NEGOTIATING THE THERAPEUTIC ALLIANCE

NEGOTIATING THE THERAPEUTIC ALLIANCE

A Relational Treatment Guide

Jeremy D. Safran
J. Christopher Muran

THE GUILFORD PRESS
New York   London

Printed in the United States of America

This book is printed on acid-free paper.

Last digit is print number: 9 8 7 6 5 4 3 2 1

Library of Congress Cataloging-in-Publication Data
available from the Publisher

ISBN 1-57230-512-6

Portions of Chapter 1 are adapted from Muran, J. C., & Safran,
J. D. (1998). Negotiating the therapeutic alliance in brief psychotherapy. In
J. D. Safran & J. C. Muran (Eds.), *The therapeutic alliance in brief
psychotherapy* (pp. 3–14). Washington, DC: American Psychological
Association Books. Copyright 1998 by the American Psychological
Association. Portions of Chapter 3 are adapted from Safran, J. D. (1999).
Faith, despair, will, and the paradox of acceptance. *Contemporary
Psychoanalysis, 35,* 5–24. Copyright 1999 by the W. A. White Institute; and
Safran, J. D. (1993). Breaches in the therapeutic alliance: An arena for
negotiating authentic relatedness. *Psychotherapy, 30,* 11–24. Copyright 1993
by *Psychotherapy* and adapted by permission of the American Psychological
Association. Chapter 6 is adapted from Safran, J. D. (in press). Brief
relational psychoanalytic treatment. *Psychoanalytic Dialogues.* Copyright by
The Analytic Press, Inc. Excerpt from "East Coker" in *Four Quartets* by T. S.
Eliot. Copyright 1940 by T. S. Eliot and renewed 1968 by Esme Valerie
Eliot, reprinted by permission of Harcourt, Inc. Excerpt from *Open Mouth
Already a Mistake, Talks by Zen Master Wu Kwang.* Copyright 1997 by Primary
Point Press. Reprinted by permission.

To Jenny—J. D. S.

To Elisa—J. C. M.

About the Authors

Jeremy D. Safran, PhD, is Professor of Psychology at the New School for Social Research, where he was formerly Director of Clinical Psychology. He is also Senior Research Scientist at New York's Beth Israel Medical Center. He is the author of *Widening the Scope of Cognitive Therapy*, coauthor of *Emotion in Psychotherapy* and *Interpersonal Process in Cognitive Therapy*, and coeditor of *Emotion, Psychotherapy, and Change* and *The Therapeutic Alliance in Brief Psychotherapy*. He is an advisory editor for *Psychotherapy Research, Journal of Clinical Psychology, Journal of Psychotherapy Integration*, and several other journals, and maintains a private practice in New York City.

J. Christopher Muran, PhD, is Chief Psychologist and Director of the Brief Psychotherapy Research Program at Beth Israel Medical Center, where he maintains a private practice. He is also Associate Professor of Psychiatry at Albert Einstein College of Medicine. He completed a fellowship in cognitive-behavioral therapy at the Clarke Institute of Psychiatry, University of Toronto, as well as analytic training in the New York University Postdoctoral Program. He received the Early Career Award from the Society for Psychotherapy Research, and serves as an advisory editor for *Psychotherapy Research*. He is coeditor of *The Therapeutic Alliance in Brief Psychotherapy* and editor of the forthcoming *Self-Relations in the Psychotherapy Process*.

Acknowledgments

The writing of this book was supported in part by Grant No. MH50246 from the National Institute of Mental Health. We would like to acknowledge the assistance of a number of people who provided valuable feedback during various stages of its development. Lewis Aron provided encouraging and perceptive comments on a number of chapters while the book was still in an early stage of development. Stanley Messer, Jeffrey Binder, and Jennifer Hunter provided detailed, thoughtful, and helpful feedback on later drafts. We would also like to express our appreciation to Arnold Winston, who has provided ongoing emotional and material support for our research program on the therapeutic alliance, and to Lisa Wallner Samstag for her ongoing collaboration. Thanks also to Seymour Weingarten and Kitty Moore at The Guilford Press. And, finally, we would like to express our appreciation to our patients and to the many therapists participating in our training groups over the years who have pushed us to continually refine our thinking.

Contents

Consider the speech of "primitive" peoples, that is, of those that have a meagre stock of objects, and whose life is built up within a narrow circle of acts highly charged with presentness. The nuclei of this speech, words in the form of sentences and original pre-grammatical structures (which later, splitting asunder, give rise to the many various kinds of words), mostly indicate wholeness in relation. We say "far away"; the Zulu has for that a word which means in our sentence form, "There where someone cries out: 'Oh mother, I am lost.' " The Fuegian soars above our analytic wisdom with a seven-syllabled word whose precise meaning is, "They stare at one another, each waiting for the other to volunteer to do what both wish, but are not able to do." In this total situation the persons, as expressed both in nouns and pronouns, are embedded, still only in relief and without finished independence. The chief concern is not with these products of analysis and reflection but with the true original unity, the lived relation.

—MARTIN BUBER

There was a monk who studied with Zen Master Ko Sahn. This monk became dissatisfied with his progress and began to travel widely to other Zen Masters and other Zen temples. But wherever he went, he was asked, "Where are you coming from?" and he replied, "From Zen Master Ko Sahn." Everyone said, "Oh, Ko Sahn, he's a very great and unusual Zen Master. You are very fortunate." Finally, the monk turned around and returned to Ko Sahn's place. He decided to interview Ko Sahn one more time. He asked the Zen Master, "You have a very special knowledge of Zen. Why is it that you never revealed it to me?" Ko Sahn said, "When you boiled rice, didn't I light the match to the fire? When you passed around the food, didn't I also hold out my bowl?" At this the monk attained enlightenment.

—TRADITIONAL ZEN TALE

At times the analyst must do everything in his power not to become, or to behave as, a separate, sharply-contoured object. In other words, he must allow his patients to relate to, or exist with him as if he were one of the primary substances. This means that he should be willing to carry the patient, not actively but like water carries the swimmer or the earth carries the walker, that is, to be there for the patient, to be used without too much resistance against being used. . . . Over and above all this, he must be there, must always be there, and must be indestructible—as are water and earth.

—MICHAEL BALINT

✳ 1

The Therapeutic Alliance Reconsidered

After approximately a half century of psychotherapy research, one of the most consistent findings is that the quality of the therapeutic alliance is the most robust predictor of treatment success. This finding has been evident across a wide range of treatment modalities (Alexander & Luborsky, 1986; Horvath, Gaston, & Luborsky, 1993; Horvath & Greenberg, 1994; Horvath & Symonds, 1991; Orlinsky, Grawe, & Parks, 1994). A related finding is that poor outcome cases show greater evidence of negative interpersonal process (i.e., hostile and complex interactions between therapists and patients) than good outcome cases (Henry, Schacht, & Strupp, 1986, 1990; Coady, 1991; Kiesler & Watkins, 1989; Tasca & McMullen, 1992; Binder & Strupp, 1997). Another related finding is that some therapists are consistently more helpful than others; differences in therapist ability seem to be more important than therapeutic modality, and the more helpful therapists appear better able to facilitate the development of a therapeutic alliance (Luborsky, McLellan, Diguer, Woody, & Seligman, 1997). A consensus is thus emerging around two related issues: that negative process and ruptures or strains in the alliance are an inevitability, and that one of the most important therapeutic skills consists of dealing therapeutically with this type of negative process and repairing ruptures in the therapeutic alliance (e.g., Bordin, 1994; Horvath, 1995; Henry & Strupp, 1994; Foreman & Marmar, 1985; Rhodes, Hill, Thompson, & Elliott, 1994; Binder & Strupp, 1997).

1

This book was written as a guide for training therapists to work constructively with negative process in psychotherapy and to skillfully negotiate ruptures in the therapeutic alliance. Two major impetuses have shaped the development of this book. The first has been our own research program on the therapeutic alliance (Safran, Crocker, McMain, & Murray, 1990; Safran, 1993a, 1993b, 1999; Safran, Muran, & Samstag, 1994; Safran & Muran, 1994, 1995, 1996, 1998; see also Muran et al., 1995; Muran, Segal, Samstag, & Crawford, 1994; Safran & Wallner, 1991). The second has been our attempts to synthesize and systematize those developments in contemporary psychotherapy theory that we find most relevant.

In terms of the first impetus, we began our research on the therapeutic alliance in the late 1980s at the Clarke Institute of Psychiatry in Toronto, studying alliance ruptures and beginning to delineate the processes and principles involved in rupture resolution. Our work continued through the 1990s at Beth Israel Medical Center in New York, where we began a pilot project funded by the National Institute of Mental Health to investigate the efficacy of a specialized treatment approach for resolving ruptures in the therapeutic alliance. This project was conceptualized as the logical next step to our previous research efforts to clarify the processes through which problems in the therapeutic alliance are successfully resolved. As part of this research project, we developed a manual for training therapists. This book evolved out of that manual.

In terms of the second impetus, we have been influenced by diverse psychotherapy traditions. These include psychoanalysis, the experiential tradition (gestalt and client-centered therapy), and cognitive therapy. Most influential, however, has been a series of related developments in contemporary psychoanalytic theory that have come to be collectively referred to as "relational theory" (Aron, 1996; Greenberg & Mitchell, 1983; Mitchell, 1988, 1993, 1997). Relational theory, itself integrative in nature, attempts to synthesize developments from such diverse areas as American interpersonal theory, British object relations theory, self psychology, existential thinking, and feminist and postmodern thinking. One of the central tenets of relational theory is that the therapist and the patient are always participating in a relational configuration that they cannot see, and the process of coming to understand and disembed from this configuration is a central mechanism of change. We find relational theory to be particularly useful for organizing insights and principles from other therapeutic traditions that are relevant to the topic of therapeutic impasses, and as such have adopted it as our overarching theoretical framework.

This book can thus be viewed as an attempt to systematize some of the central principles of relational thinking in psychoanalysis. In this respect, it can be thought of as an update to the manuals written by Hans Strupp and Jeffrey Binder (1984) and Lester Luborsky (1984) in the mid-1980s. Both of these books did superb jobs of systematizing some of the major developments in psychoanalytic theory as of that time for training purposes. Since that time, however, there has been what many people think of as a paradigm shift in psychoanalytic thinking, along relational lines. Some of the developments that have taken place were outlined by Hanna Levenson (1995) in her elaboration of Strupp and Binder's approach. She was more concerned, however, with refining and teaching their approach than with manualizing relational psychoanalytic thinking. Many of these recent developments, however, are particularly useful for shedding light on how to deal with problems in the therapeutic alliance. Consequently, it seems important to systematize some of these newer theoretical and technical developments into a manualized form.

The mid- to late 1980s were marked by considerable enthusiasm among psychotherapists about the role that treatment manuals could potentially play in facilitating the training of therapists (e.g., Luborsky & DeRubeis, 1984; Strupp, Butler, & Rosser, 1988). Many felt that the precise specification of treatment principles and techniques characteristic of treatment manuals, by identifying the critical therapeutic skills in an unambiguous fashion, should be able to translate into improvements in clinical practice. Although there continues to be enthusiasm about the value of treatment manuals (e.g., Wilson, 1998; Heimberg, 1998; Barlow, 1996), many have become less optimistic (e.g., Goldfried & Wolfe, 1998; Lambert, 1998; Henry, 1998; Seligman, 1995). The consistent finding is that treatment manual adherence does not relate to treatment outcome (e.g., Moncher & Prinz, 1991). Critics argue that treatment manuals artificially constrain the clinical practice of therapists and reduce treatment flexibility and therapist creativity.

Some of the more interesting and systematic research on the influence of manualized training on treatment process and outcome has been conducted by Hans Strupp and his colleagues (Henry, Schacht, Strupp, Butler, & Binder, 1993; Henry, Strupp, Butler, Schacht, & Binder, 1993; Strupp, 1993). In the Vanderbilt II study, experienced therapists treated a first cohort of patients and were subsequently given a full year's intensive training in a manualized form of psychodynamic treatment that places special emphasis on the detection and management of maladaptive interpersonal patterns with particular emphasis on their enactment within the therapeutic relationship. The therapists then treated a second cohort of patients, and differences in therapy process and outcome following training were evaluated.

Although therapists, following the training period, were observed to work in a way that more closely corresponded to the treatment manual (e.g., focusing on the patient–therapist relationship and addressing transactions in the here-and-now), these differences did not necessarily translate into more skillful therapy. In fact, the therapists were actually found to display more evidence of negative process with their patients in the form of hostile interactions or complex communications (i.e., interpretations that are at one level helpful and at another level critical). Of particular interest was the finding that therapists who were assessed as more self-controlling and self-blaming were more likely to adhere to the treatment manual and more likely to display negative process (less warmth and friendliness and more hostility) with their patients. They also tended to have the poorest outcomes. Thus, as Hans Strupp and Timothy Anderson (1997) concluded, the training process was filtered through the therapists' preexisting personality dispositions. Furthermore, Strupp and his colleagues observed that in general therapists tended to deliver the manualized treatment interventions in a fairly forced mechanical fashion, and that they never came to feel comfortable or natural with them (Henry, Strupp, et al., 1993). The treatment approach continued to be experienced as an outside standard that they were trying to conform to, rather than as a personally integrated way of being-in-the-room with patients. Findings of this type raise important questions about how best to conceptualize the expertise possessed by skilled therapists and how to facilitate acquiring such expertise.

One reason that it is so difficult to train psychotherapists is that the acquisition of therapeutic skill is, as Strupp and his colleagues' findings suggest, mediated by complex personal and emotional factors. Growth as therapists is thus inextricably tied to personal growth and the development of self-awareness. A second factor is that therapeutic skill has important intuitive and creative aspects to it that are difficult (if not impossible) to teach. Research on the nature of professional expertise makes it clear that highly skilled practitioners across a range of fields respond to relevant situations in a flexible, creative, and contextually sensitive fashion (Dreyfus & Dreyfus, 1986; Schon, 1983). Unlike novices, who tend to apply rules in a "cookbook" type of manner, experts engage in what Schon (1983) refers to as *reflection-in-action*. This involves treating new cases as unique and constructing new theories to fit them, rather than depending on categories of established theory and technique. This does not mean that existing theory and technique are irrelevant, but rather that they are elaborated, refined, and modified through ongoing "conversation" with the existing situation.

The task that we set for ourselves in developing the current treatment guide was to create a resource to facilitate the development of this type of reflection-in-action, rather than a cookbook that would lend itself to a type of mechanical implementation. To this end, we have incorporated a number of features. The first is that we have tried to strike a balance between writing at a concrete technical level that is more prescriptive in nature and writing at a more general theoretical level that conveys the essence of the approach. In this way, we hope to avoid the pitfalls of, at one extreme, writing a narrowly technical manual that constrains therapists and interferes with creativity, and, at the other extreme, writing an abstract treatise that is not linked to practical specifics.

A second feature is that we place considerable emphasis on the inner work of the therapist. Many therapeutic orientations assume that the therapist's personal growth is important; indeed, the analysis of countertransference is at the heart of contemporary psychoanalytic technique. Despite this fact, systematic attempts to spell out the internal processes involved in harnessing and working constructively with the intense, conflictual, and often painful feelings and thoughts that emerge for therapists when negotiating difficult moments with patients are rare. Unless the therapist has the ability to engage in this type of inner work, however, his or her conceptual grasp of relevant theoretical and technical principles is useless.

A third feature is that we place considerable emphasis on training. One of the major conclusions emerging from the Vanderbilt II study and from our own experience is that training therapists to deal with negative process in psychotherapy and therapeutic impasses is a formidable task. A failure to explore training issues in depth, therefore, would be a serious omission in a book such as this one. Because of the complexity of the skills therapists require to deal with negative therapeutic process, it is critical for their training to be more experiential in nature and to emphasize self-exploration as a primary vehicle for learning. Because of the importance of this topic, we have devoted an entire chapter to it.

Finally, we have illustrated the major principles with extensive transcript material. We view this to be a critical part of the process of grounding the more theoretical aspects of the book in concrete specifics and providing therapists with clear illustrations of how they can be implemented in practice.

OVERVIEW OF THE BOOK

This book begins with more general theoretical considerations and then moves toward outlining principles of a more specific and technical nature. The rest of Chapter 1 continues with a discussion of the history of the concept of the therapeutic alliance and a reconceptualiztion of the concept that is in keeping with contemporary theoretical perspectives. It concludes with a taxonomy of principles for negotiating problems in the therapeutic alliance.

Chapter 2 (Fundamental Assumptions and Principles) outlines a number of assumptions and principles that provide a foundation for purposes of orienting therapists in the "right" direction. In this chapter we attempt to convey the essence of our approach (i.e., values and ways of viewing things that seem most important). Most of these principles are of a more general nature in that they are relevant to psychotherapy practice as a whole. At the same time, however, they have important implications for working through therapeutic impasses.

Chapter 3 (Understanding Alliance Ruptures and Therapeutic Impasses) focuses specifically on theoretical issues that are more directly relevant to the topic of therapeutic impasses. We outline a range of complementary theories and points of view that can provide useful frameworks for thinking about alliance ruptures and the processes involved in working through them constructively.

Chapters 4 and 5 are more technical in nature. Chapter 4 (Therapeutic Metacommunication: Mindfulness in Action) outlines various principles to guide the process of collaboratively exploring and working through therapeutic impasses with patients. The focus in this chapter is on general and specific principles of metacommunication (i.e., the process of making explicit what is being unwittingly enacted in the therapeutic relationship). Chapter 5 (Stage-Process Models of Alliance Rupture Resolution) examines the interactional patterns that are characteristic of therapist–patient dyads who are able to successfully negotiate therapeutic alliance ruptures. This chapter is based on our research program on the topic.

Chapter 6 (Brief Relational Therapy) applies the principles outlined in the previous chapters to short-term therapy. It also provides an extensive case illustration (with transcript material) of a patient treated with this approach. Finally, Chapter 7 (Training and Supervision) spells out the central principles outlining our training approach and illustrates them with a transcript of a training session. These final two chapters have also been influenced substantially by our research program.

A BRIEF HISTORY OF THE THERAPEUTIC ALLIANCE

The importance of the therapeutic relationship was originally discussed by Sigmund Freud in his early theoretical papers on transference. Although he first spoke of making a "collaborator" of the patient in the therapeutic process (Breuer & Freud, 1893–1895), Freud (1912) was primarily concerned with the transferential aspects of the relationship and the importance of transference analysis. For Freud, *transference* involved the displacement of affects from one object or person to another, most often the transference of attitudes formerly associated with a parent. He distinguished between positive and negative transferences (i.e., the transference of positive versus negative attitudes). Freud also spoke of the "unobjectionable positive transference," the aspect of the transference that should not be analyzed because it provides the patient with the motivation necessary to collaborate effectively with the analyst. To a limited extent he did acknowledge the role of friendliness and affection as "the vehicle of success in psychoanalysis" (Freud, 1912) and suggested that the analyst and patient must band together against the patient's symptoms in an "analytic pact" based on free exploration by the patient and competent understanding by the analyst (Freud, 1937, 1940).

From Freud, one can trace the development of psychoanalytic perspectives on the therapeutic relationship to two emergent lines. The first developed through the influence of Sandor Ferenczi (see Aron & Harris, 1991). As analyst to Balint, Jones, Klein, and Rickman, he had a great impact on British object relations theory. As analyst to Thompson, Roheim, and Rado, Ferenczi likewise influenced interpersonal and cultural psychoanalysis in America. Ferenczi (1932) was the first to suggest that it was essential for patients not merely to remember but actually to relive the problematic past in the therapeutic relationship. Thus he sowed ideas later cultivated by Michael Balint (1968), D. W. Winnicott (1965), and Franz Alexander (with his notion of the corrective emotional experience; see Alexander & French, 1946). Ferenczi was also the first to consider the role of the analyst's personality and experience in the treatment process. He highlighted the analyst as a real person and recognized the real impact of the analyst on the transference–countertransference enactment (Ferenczi, 1932). Thus he suggested ideas developed further by the interpersonalists, such as participant-observation (Thompson, 1944).

The second line can be identified as the ego psychological tradition, which emphasized the reality-oriented adaptation of the ego to its environment (A. Freud, 1936; Hartmann, 1958). Partially in response to the exclusive view held particularly by Kleinians that all meaningful reactions of the patient to the person of the analyst are transference manifestations and that the only important interventions are transference interpretations, the ego analysts refocused attention on the real aspects of the therapeutic relationship and developed the notion of the working or therapeutic alliance (Greenson, 1971). The concept of the alliance was the ego psychological attempt to bring the interaction between analyst and patient to the fore. It permitted modifications in the traditional analytic stance and the use of noninterpretive measures; moreover, it encouraged greater technical flexibility and enabled the adaption of analytic techniques for a wider range of patients. By introducing the alliance concept, the ego psychologists were also attempting to resolve the Freudian paradox that the analyst uses transference to enable the patient to overcome transference (Friedman, 1969; Meissner, 1996).

Richard Sterba (1934, 1940) helped establish the groundwork on which the alliance concept was developed. He was the first to explicate the role of positive identification with the therapist in leading the patient to work toward the accomplishment of common therapeutic tasks. Sterba spoke about the importance of helping the patient to form a "therapeutic split in the ego" between its observant and participant functions so that the reality-focused elements of the ego could become allied with the therapist in the task of self-observation. His was an effort to split rationality and irrationality. Otto Fenichel (1941) described Sterba's conceptualization of the alliance as the "rational transference," while Leo Stone (1961) referred to it as the "mature transference."

It was Elizabeth Zetzel (1956, 1966) who first formally argued that the therapeutic alliance is essential to the effectiveness of any therapeutic intervention (crediting the term to E. Bibring, 1937). She argued that the alliance is dependent on the patient's fundamental capacity to form a stable trusting relationship, which in turn is rooted in his or her early developmental experiences. She believed that when this capacity does not exist at the outset, it is critical for the therapist to provide a supportive relationship that facilitates the development of an alliance, in the same way that a mother needs to provide the appropriate maternal environment to facilitate the development of a fundamental sense of trust.

Lawrence Friedman (1969) similarly adopted a maternal model for the alliance, emphasizing the roles of rapport and hope. He viewed the alliance as encompassing both rational and irrational elements, including the more infantile maternal transference. Likewise, Phyllis Greenacre (1968) and Joseph Sandler and colleagues (Sandler, Holder, Kawenoka, Kennedy, & Neurath, 1969) linked the notion of the "basic or primary transference" to the alliance concept. This perspective bears some resemblance to the use of the therapist-as-mother metaphor in British object relations conceptualizations of the psychotherapeutic process; for example, both the Winnicottian (Winnicott, 1965) notion of "holding environment" and the Kleinian (Bion, 1962) notion of "containment" assume this type of maternal metaphor.

Ralph Greenson (1967, 1971) extended the ego psychological tradition with a seminal formulation of the therapeutic relationship. He described this relationship as consisting of a transference configuration and a real relationship (although he recognized that the boundary is somewhat artificial). The *real relationship* refers to the mutual human response of the patient and therapist to each other, including undistorted perceptions and authentic liking, trust, and respect for each other. Greenson conceptualized the working alliance as the ability of the patient and therapist to work purposefully together in the treatment they have undertaken. Although the patient's transference reactions may support the working alliance, the essential core of the alliance is the real relationship. By making such a distinction, Greenson, like Sterba before him, emphasized the importance of rationality and objectivity in therapy.

Over the years, many have grappled with the questions of how to conceptualize the relationship between the alliance and transferential aspects of the therapeutic relationship and whether the alliance concept is meaningful and useful (e.g., Dickes, 1975; Kanzer, 1975; Langs, 1976). Charles Brenner (1979), for example, argued that it is meaningless to distinguish between alliance and transference since all aspects of the patient's relationship to the therapist are determined by past experiences. From his perspective, the danger of the alliance concept is that it can lead therapists to leave aspects of the transference unanalyzed and promote an emphasis on change through suggestion rather than through understanding. Homer Curtis (1979) followed Brenner in cautioning that the alliance concept may lead therapists to label some aspects of the therapeutic relationship as "realistic" and therefore not to be analyzed. This, he believed, might lead therapists to fail to explore the conflictual motivation that might lie beneath the patient's positive feelings toward the therapist. Unlike Brenner, however, he did not recommend completely discarding the alliance concept, and he did emphasize the importance of recognizing the fundamental importance of the patient's trust in and cooperation with the therapist. Jacques Lacan (1973a, 1973b), consistent with his critique of American ego analysis, viewed the idea of an alliance between the therapist and a rational part of the patient's psyche as promoting a type of conformity with the desire of the other. Charles Hanly (1992) argued that the alliance concept can lead to an overvaluation of the role played by conscious, rational processes in therapy and a failure to recognize the importance of unconscious processes. Echoing Brenner, he maintained that, insofar as the concept of the alliance implies an independence from transference, it may lead therapists to emphasize the "human influence" of the therapeutic relationship at the expense of the search for correct interpretations.

Among American interpersonalists (e.g., Lionells, Fiscalini, Mann, & Stern, 1995), the alliance concept has not received much attention (see Fiscalini, 1988; Gutheil & Havens, 1979, for exceptions). There are a number of reasons for this. First, the interpersonal tradition never adopted the classical analytic prescriptions of therapist neutrality and abstinence. There has thus always been more room for technical flexibility. Moreover, from the outset, Harry Stack Sullivan was exquisitely attuned to subtle fluctuations in the patient's anxiety level and particularly concerned about the importance of keeping this anxiety at a manageable level in order to avoid a disintegration of the therapist–patient relationship. In a sense, then, he was implicitly concerned with the skillful management of the alliance, and the formal development and refinement of the concept was not critical. Second, there has always been an important thread in the interpersonal tradition that emphasizes the therapist's ultimate embeddedness in the interpersonal field and his or her irreducible subjectivity (e.g., Stern, 1997). Sullivan, despite his introduction of field theory and the notion of the participant-observer, believed that the therapist could to some extent stand outside of the interpersonal field and maintain the stance of the expert. Subsequent interpersonal theorists, however, moved toward a more radical perspective that challenged any notion of therapist objectivity (e.g., Levenson, 1992). Moreover, from the beginning, both Sullivan and Clara Thompson (1964) emphasized the importance of the real relationship between therapist and patient. Related to this, Erich Fromm (1947) played an important role in emphasizing the importance of the existential encounter as a vehicle of change. For all of these reasons, there has been less of a need to explicitly formulate the concept of the therapeutic alliance.

Recent developments in contemporary psychoanalytic theory toward a relational perspective (e.g., Mitchell, 1988) have extended the interpersonal emphasis on therapist participation and subjectivity. These developments include perspectives influenced by feminist theory, social constructivist discourse, and the notion of intersubjectivity (see Aron, 1996). Relational thinking opposes the rigid demarcation between subject and object, between observer and observed, with its emphasis on reason and rationality. What is real or unreal, true or untrue, is replaced by the recognition that there are multiple truths and that these truths are socially constructed. The distinction between transference and real aspects of the relationship thus becomes meaningless. The classical psychoanalytic emphasis on neutrality, anonymity, and abstinence has given way to an emphasis on "interaction, enactment, spontaneity, mutuality, and authenticity" (Mitchell, 1997, p. ix). It is probably for these reasons that the concept of the alliance receives less theoretical attention these days in psychoanalytic circles than it did at one time (with some notable exceptions, e.g., Meissner, 1996; Wallerstein, 1995), although most analysts still take it for granted as a necessary component of the process.

At the same time, the concept of the alliance has spread to other therapeutic traditions, where it is increasingly accorded central status. While the quality of the therapeutic relationship has always been seen as a central curative agent in the experiential tradition (e.g., Rogers, 1951, 1957), contemporary experiential theorists (e.g., Greenberg, Rice, & Elliott, 1993) have explicitly adopted the concept of the alliance. They have found that as they integrate an empathic stance with more directive interventions, the concept of the alliance becomes particularly useful. While the cognitive-behavioral perspective traditionally paid less importance to the therapeutic relationship, contemporary cognitive-behavioral theorists are increasingly recognizing the central importance of the alliance (e.g., Arnkoff, 1995; Goldfried & Davison, 1974, 1994; Kohlenberg & Tsai, 1991; Muran, 1993; Muran & Ventur, 1995; Newman, 1998; Safran, 1998; Safran & Segal, 1990). Similar trends are emerging in family therapy (e.g., Pinsof & Catherall, 1986; Rait, 1998), group therapy (e.g., Mackenzie, 1998), and strategic therapy (e.g., Coyne & Pepper, 1998).

As Wolfe and Goldfried (1988) maintain, the therapeutic alliance is the "quintessential integrative variable." The growing recognition by diverse therapeutic traditions of the importance of the therapeutic alliance can be attributed, at least in part, to its centrality in the psychotherapy research community (e.g., Horvath & Greenberg, 1994; Horvath & Luborsky, 1993), where there has been a proliferation of measures and evidence demonstrating the predictive validity of the concept (Gaston, 1990; Hartley, 1985; Horvath & Symonds, 1991). Interest in this concept among researchers can be partly attributed to the search for understanding change across treatments, given that no particular treatment has been shown to be consistently more effective than any other (Smith, Glass, & Miller, 1980). It was also catalyzed by the early empirical work of Lester Luborsky (1976) and by Edward Bordin (1979), who attracted considerable attention within the psychotherapy research community with his transtheoretical reformulation of the alliance concept. Bordin suggested that a good alliance is a prerequisite for change in all forms of psychotherapy. He conceptualized the alliance as consisting of three interdependent components: tasks, goals, and the bond. According to him, the strength of the alliance is dependent on the degree of agreement between patient and therapist about the tasks and goals of therapy, and on the quality of the relational bond between them.

The *tasks of therapy* consist of the specific activities (either overt or covert) that the patient must engage in to benefit from the treatment. For example, classical psychoanalysis requires the patient to try to free-associate by attempting to say whatever comes to mind without censoring it. An important task in cognitive therapy may consist of completing a behavioral assignment between sessions. Gestalt therapists may ask their patients to engage in a dialogue between two different parts of the self.

The *goals of therapy* are the general objectives toward which the treatment is directed. For example, classical psychoanalysis assumes that the problems that bring people into therapy result from a maladaptive way of negotiating the conflict between instincts and defenses, and the goal consists of developing a more adaptive way of negotiating that conflict. A behavior therapist, in contrast, may see the goal of treatment as one of removing a specific symptom.

The *bond* component of the alliance consists of the affective quality of the relationship between patient and therapist (e.g., the extent to which the patient feels understood, respected, valued, and so on). The bond, task, and goal dimensions of the alliance influence one another in an ongoing fashion. The quality of the bond mediates the extent to which the patient and the therapist are able to negotiate an agreement about the tasks and goals of therapy, and the ability to negotiate an agreement about the tasks and goals in therapy in turn mediates the quality of the bond.

Thus, Bordin's conceptualization highlights the complex, dynamic, and multidimensional nature of the alliance. It suggests that while the quality of the alliance is critical in all therapeutic approaches, the specific variables mediating this quality will vary as a function of a complex, interdependent, and fluctuating matrix of therapist, patient, and approach-specific features. Bordin's conceptualization is therefore a rich and deceptively simple concept that highlights the fundamental independence of therapy-specific (i.e., technical) and nonspecific (i.e., relational) factors (Safran, 1993b).

A RECONCEPTUALIZATION
OF THE THERAPEUTIC ALLIANCE

Historically, the concept of the therapeutic alliance has played an important role in the evolution of the classical psychoanalytic tradition, insofar as it has provided a theoretical justification for greater technical flexibility. By highlighting the critical importance of the real, human aspects of the therapeutic relationship, it has provided grounds for departing from the idealized therapist stance of abstinence and neutrality. With the growing ascendance of relational thinking (e.g., Aron, 1996; Mitchell, 1988, 1993, 1997), the question arises as to whether the concept of the alliance is still valuable. Interpersonal and relational perspectives do not adhere to classical notions of therapist abstinence and neutrality and provide considerably more scope for technical flexibility. Moreover, from these perspectives, the experience of a constructive relational experience with the therapist is viewed as a critical component of change. In fact, one might say that the processes of developing and resolving problems in alliance are not the prerequisites to change, but rather the very essence of the change process.

Nevertheless, we believe that a broadened conceptualization of the therapeutic alliance along the lines that Bordin has suggested is still useful for several reasons. First, it highlights the fact that at a fundamental level the patient's ability to trust, hope, and have faith in the therapist's ability to help always plays a central role in the change process. Some aspects of the alliance may involve conscious, rational deliberation, but other aspects are unconscious and affectively based. Second, it highlights the fact that different types of alliance are necessary depending on the relevant therapeutic tasks and goals. The type of alliance focused on by such theorists as Greenson and Sterba, which emphasizes the patient's rational collaboration with the therapist on the task of self-observation, is only one type of alliance.

There are a wide range of other therapeutic tasks and goals both within psychoanalysis and within other forms of psychotherapy; for example, accessing painful feelings or reconstructing historical memories (psychoanalysis), monitoring and recording one's internal dialogue between sessions (cognitive therapy), and engaging in a dialogue between different parts of the self (gestalt therapy). The process of relating to the therapist in an authentic and organismically grounded fashion (common to both existential and relational psychoanalytic approaches) can be thought of as yet another therapeutic task.

Each of these tasks places different demands on patients and will tend to be experienced by them as more or less helpful depending upon their own capacities and characteristic ways of relating to themselves and others (Bordin, 1979, 1994; Safran, 1993a, 1993b). One patient may find the task of exploring emotional experience especially difficult. Another may find the task of exploring the therapeutic relationship in the here-and-now as particularly difficult. Still another may experience structured cognitive-behavioral exercises as reassuring and containing. Another may experience a therapist's suggestion to do homework between sessions as controlling or domineering.

This broadened conceptualization of the alliance has a number of important implications. First, it highlights the interdependence of relational and technical factors in psychotherapy. It suggests that the meaning of any technical factor can only be understood in the relational context in which it is applied. Any intervention may have a positive or a negative impact on the quality of the bond between the patient and the therapist depending on its idiosyncratic meaning to the patient, and conversely any intervention may be experienced as more or less facilitative depending on the preexisting bond.

Second, it provides a framework for guiding the therapist's interventions in a flexible fashion. Rather than basing one's approach on some inflexible and idealized criterion such as therapeutic neutrality, one can be guided by an understanding of what a particular therapeutic task means to a particular patient in a given moment. How is an exploratory question experienced by the patient? Does it facilitate greater understanding of an issue? Does it close off an exploration because it feels intrusive or it evokes too much anxiety to tolerate? How is a given interpretation experienced? Is it experienced as empathic or critical? Is the abstinent stance of a classical analyst experienced as withholding or respectful? Is the client-centered therapist's reluctance to make interpretations experienced as empathic or abandoning? Are Kleinian interpretations experienced as invasive or empathic? Are rational-emotive confrontations experienced as respectful or invalidating?

Third, as Robert Stolorow and colleagues (Stolorow, Brandchaft, & Atwood, 1994) have highlighted, ruptures in the therapeutic alliance are the royal road to understanding the patient's core organizing principles. As contemporary Kleinians, such as Betty Joseph (1989), point out, the therapist should attend on an ongoing basis to the way in which patients respond to her interventions. The exploration of the factors underlying the patient's construal of an intervention as hindering can provide a rich understanding of the patient's idiosyncratic construal processes and internal object relations.

Fourth, this conceptualization of the alliance highlights the importance of the *negotiation* between patient and therapist about the tasks and goals of therapy. More traditional conceptualizations of the alliance assume that there is only one therapeutic task (i.e., rational collaboration with the therapist in the task of self-observation), or at least privilege this task over others. Although Sterba, Zetzel, and Greenson emphasized the importance of the therapist acting in a supportive fashion in order to facilitate the development of the alliance, ultimately they assumed that the patient will identify with the therapist and adapt to the therapist's conceptualization of the tasks and goals of therapy or accept the therapist's understanding of the value of these tasks and goals. In contrast, Bordin's conceptualization of the alliance is more dynamic and mutual. It assumes that there will be an ongoing negotiation between therapist and patient at both conscious and unconscious levels about the tasks and goals of therapy and that this process of negotiation both establishes the necessary conditions for change to take place and is an intrinsic part of the change process.

This conceptualization of the alliance as entailing an ongoing negotiation is consistent with an increasingly influential way of conceptualizing the therapeutic process in contemporary relational thinking. Jessica Benjamin (1990) was one of the first to argue that the process of negotiation between two different subjectivities is at the heart of the change process. Stephen Mitchell (1993) emphasizes that the negotiation between the patient's desires and those of the therapist is a critical therapeutic mechanism. Stuart Pizer (1992) also describes the essence of therapeutic action as constituted by the engagement of two persons in a process of negotiation. He suggests that therapists in their interventions and patients in their responses are recurrently saying to each other, "No, you can't make this of me. But you can make that of me" (1992, p. 218). Pizer includes in this process all aspects of therapy, including the agreement on fees, the arrangement about scheduling, and so on. He argues that "the very substances and nature of truth and reality . . . are being negotiated toward consensus" in the therapeutic relationship (1992, p. 218).

This line of thought deepens our understanding of the significance of the negotiation between therapists and patients about therapeutic tasks and goals. It suggests that this process is not only about a superficial negotiation toward consensus. At a deeper level, it taps into fundamental dilemmas of human existence, such as the negotiation of one's desires with those of another, the struggle to experience oneself as a subject while at the same time recognizing the subjectivity of the other, and the tension between the need for agency versus the need for relatedness. We will elaborate on these themes in the coming chapter.

A TAXONOMY OF INTERVENTIONS
FOR ADDRESSING ALLIANCE RUPTURES

The skilled clinician uses a wide range of different interventions for building and managing the therapeutic alliance and working through ruptures in the alliance as they develop. While some of the principles guiding these interventions are spelt out explicitly in the various theories that guide practitioners of diverse orientations (e.g., analyzing the transference in psychoanalysis or outlining the treatment rationale in cognitive-behavioral therapy), others are more implicit in nature; that is, they constitute part of what is typically referred to as the "nonspecific aspect" of psychotherapy. In this section, we outline a taxonomy for purposes of organizing our thinking about the range of possible interventions that can be employed for negotiating the therapeutic alliance and dealing with treatment impasses resulting from strains in the alliance. In subsequent chapters we will elaborate on some of the more important interventions and underlying principles in greater detail.

Following Bordin's (1979) conceptualization of the alliance, we find it useful to conceptualize ruptures in the alliance as consisting either of *disagreements* about the *tasks* or *goals* of therapy or of *problems* in the *bond* dimension (bearing in mind that disagreements about therapeutic tasks or goals often reflect strains in the bond dimension and vice versa). Each of these two types of ruptures can be addressed either *directly* or *indirectly*. For example, if a patient questions the relevance of exploring his emotions, the therapist may respond directly by providing a therapeutic rationale or indirectly by changing the therapeutic task (see Figure 1.1).

In some cases, the therapist may deal with alliance ruptures at a surface level, while in other cases the focus may be on the level of underlying meaning. For example, a disagreement about the task of therapy (e.g., reporting whatever comes to mind) can be explored in its own terms (e.g., discussing the rationale underlying the task) or in terms of an underlying relational theme (e.g., the patient feels pressured to conform, which is a common theme in his relationships with others). Although much of this book focuses on interventions targeted at the level of underlying meaning, it is important not to lose sight of the importance of focusing on the surface level as well. In everyday practice, many of the most important alliance-building or alliance-repairing interventions are directed to the surface level. For example, without giving it much conscious thought, but intuitively gauging that it will have a positive impact on the alliance, a therapist may answer a patient's questions about the purpose of an intervention or apologize for a mistake.

Interventions targeted at the surface level ultimately also have an impact at the level of underlying meaning. For example, the process of dealing with patients' concerns by providing a rationale for a particular therapeutic task not only strengthens the alliance sufficiently to encourage them to engage in the task, it also conveys at a metalevel that the therapist takes their concerns seriously enough to be willing to try and clarify the rationale. Over time, multiple instances of this type can have an impact on the fundamental way in which patients construe self–other interactions.

Disagreements on Tasks and Goals

Direct Focus on Tasks and Goals

Therapeutic Rationale and Microprocessing Tasks. One of the more basic interventions for addressing alliance ruptures consists of outlining or reiterating the treatment rationale. When therapists detect strains in the alliance, they can check to see if patients are clear about the rationale, and if not, they can reiterate it and clarify any misunderstanding. In the same vein, therapists can employ microprocessing tasks, which consist of exercises assigned to patients in order to help them develop a concrete understanding of the type of internal processes that play a role in therapeutic change (see Watson & Greenberg, 1995). For example, patients in experiential therapy can be encouraged to try *focusing* exercises (Gendlin, 1994) as a way of helping them to learn to attend to bodily-felt experience. Patients in cognitive therapy can be asked to report on their automatic thoughts in session as a way of helping them learn to self-monitor. Marsha Linehan (1992) employs mindfulness exercises to help borderline patients learn to observe, regulate, and tolerate their emotional experience.

Although conveying a therapeutic rationale to the patient is accorded a central role in the cognitive-behavioral tradition, it is typically given less emphasis in other traditions. Notable exceptions are Paul Gray (1994) and Lester Luborsky (1984) in the psychoanalytic tradition and Leslie Greenberg, Laura Rice, and Robert Elliott (1995) in the experiential tradition. Gray (1994) emphasizes the importance of explicitly educating patients about two different kinds of self-observation. The first corresponds to the traditional analytic task of free association. He instructs patients to "strive to set aside reasonable and moral judgment, permit a flow of inner spontaneity, and observe and put into

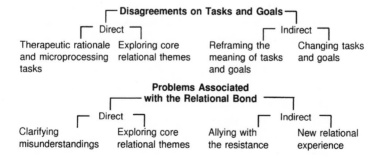

FIGURE 1.1. Therapeutic alliance rupture intervention strategies.

words unreservedly 'what comes to mind'—think out loud" (p. 67). The second consists of *retrospective self-reflection,* that is, thinking back about their own just completed mental activity, in an attempt to observe defensive processes. Luborsky (1984) provides elaborate guidelines for educating patients about psychoanalytic treatment. These involve emphasizing the importance of saying what comes to mind, discussing the concept of transference, anticipating issues such as the fact that the therapist won't give advice, and the occurrence of negative transference. Moreover, in his approach, developing an explicit core conflictual relationship theme formulation is part of the process of facilitating an agreement about the goals of treatment. Greenberg, Rice, and Elliott (1995) emphasize the importance of working to understand patients' views of their goals and of not imposing goals on them. They also emphasize the importance of educating patients about the nature of specific therapeutic tasks they may encounter, as well as the underlying rationales. Examples of such tasks include exploring and expressing unarticulated feelings and expressing different partial aspects of the self by "talking to the empty chair."

Bordin's (1979) emphasis on the importance of the task and goal dimensions of the alliance, however, highlights the critical role that the explicit discussion of the tasks and goals of therapy play in developing and maintaining a therapeutic alliance. In general, it is useful for therapists to begin treatment by exploring patients' preconceptions about how therapy works and what the therapeutic process involves, as well as their hopes regarding what will be accomplished in therapy. In situations where there is an apparent disagreement from the outset between patient and therapist about either the tasks or goals of therapy, an attempt can be made to explicitly negotiate these differences. If this attempt proves to be unsuccessful, it may be advisable to refer the patient to another therapist. For example, if a patient has a clear idea that he wants therapy to involve behavioral assignments between sessions, and the therapist is clear that she sees no role for this type of work in her approach and it looks like there is little chance of negotiating on agreement, it may be appropriate to refer a patient to someone whose approach provides a better fit to the patient.

After inquiring into the patient's preconceptions about the way in which therapy works (the tasks of therapy), it is often useful for the therapist to provide a brief description of what the work of therapy is likely to consist of, and then gauge the patient's reactions and ask whether he or she has any questions. If the patient appears not to understand or responds in a skeptical fashion, the therapist can attempt to spend some time clarifying ambiguities or addressing skepticism at the surface level by attempting to address concerns with further information or clarification. If the patient's confusion or skepticism persists, however, the therapist should try not to get locked into an interactional cycle in which he or she plays the role of the proponent attempting to convince the skeptic.

It is important for the therapist to distinguish between a genuine lack of understanding on the patient's part and an apparent confusion that reflects an underlying skepticism or mistrust. When the failure to understand a therapeutic rationale reflects an underlying skepticism or mistrust, it is important to encourage the patient to articulate whatever concerns, attitudes, or preconceptions underlie the skepticism or apparent confusion. This process can be extremely useful in terms of helping patients to begin to acknowledge whatever feelings of skepticism or mistrust they have about therapy and/or the therapist at the outset, thereby putting these attitudes into the interpersonal arena in which they can begin to be addressed.

Richard sought treatment because of a long-standing history of mild depression. He had no previous experience with therapy. In the first session the therapist asked him if he had any expectations about what would take place in treatment, and Richard replied that he did not. The therapist then proceeded to outline a brief rationale at a level that she thought would be meaningful to Richard. She explained that as a result of previous learning experiences people develop self-defeating ways of perceiving things and of relating to other people and that an important goal of treatment is to help them become aware of these self-defeating ways of being. Richard replied that he didn't understand how this would help him change. In response, the therapist indicated that many of these self-defeating ways of being operate at an automatic or unconscious level and that the process of "shining a light on them" begins to allow people choice in their lives, where previously they had none. "How are you going to shine a light?," asked Richard. "In various ways," responded his therapist. "Sometimes I may direct your attention to something you're thinking or feeling, but aren't fully aware of. Other times we may explore something going on in our relationship that may provide a clue as to things that go on in your relationships with other people." "I don't know," said Richard, "I think I'm pretty self-aware already." At this point, his therapist became aware of a feeling of futility and frustration on her part and stopped herself from continuing to persuade Richard. Instead, she began to comment on the process. "I'm aware of myself starting to get locked into trying to persuade you of something, but I have a feeling that I'm not going to be able to. It sounds to me like you're feeling kind of skeptical. Is that true?" In response, Richard was able to tentatively acknowledge some degree of skepticism, and his therapist asked him to elaborate. This led into an exploration of underlying feelings of skepticism and mistrust and a hopelessness about the possibility of changing.

In terms of the goals of therapy, it is similarly important for therapists to work with patients at the outset to help them to articulate what their goals are for the treatment. The objective here is not to establish a set of unchangeable goals that will guide the treatment from beginning to end, but rather to initiate a dialogue about goals from the outset and to ensure that the patient and therapist are on the same wavelength. This is typically accomplished by a combination of explicitly asking patients what they would like to work on and reflecting back to them an understanding of what they might want to work on in treatment, based upon those things that are both explicit and implicit in what they have said. This provides therapists with the opportunity to refine their own empathic understanding of the patient's concerns by making their provisional understanding explicit and then modifying it in light of feedback from the patient. It also helps to establish and strengthen the alliance by helping patients to feel understood and demonstrating to them that their therapist is on the same wavelength.

Over time, patients' and therapists' understanding of what the goals of therapy are will evolve through dialogue in an organic fashion. As therapy proceeds, it is important for the therapist to be vigilant for any strains in the alliance that emerge and to anticipate sensitive areas and events that might lead to such strains. For example, a therapist who has not yet explicitly explored what is being enacted in the therapeutic relationship, may prepare the way for this type of work by saying something like "I'd like to spend a little bit of time trying to understand what's going on between us right now. My hope is that this type of exploration may provide us with some clues as to what may go on for you in your relationships with other people. Does that make any sense to you?" Likewise, a therapist may pave the way for exploring the patient's defensive process by saying something like "Did you have any awareness of doing anything to interfere with your emotional experience just now? I'm going to try to direct your attention to what's going on inside at moments like this in order to help you become more aware of things that you're doing at an automatic level."

Understanding Task and Goal Disagreements in Terms of Core Relational Themes. In some situations the process of clarifying factors leading to disagreement about the tasks or goals of therapy will lead to the exploration of core relational themes for the patient. For example, a patient may experience the therapist's questions about his inner experience as intrusive, and this intrusive feeling may be related to a characteristic experience of not having his privacy respected. Another patient may have difficulty experiencing any interpretations as helpful, and this may relate to a more generalized sensitivity about feeling misunderstood by others or a readiness to feel patronized. A patient who has been sexually abused may experience the task of talking about her sexual feelings as sexually exploitative. A patient who fails to do homework assignments in cognitive therapy may have a particular sensitivity to feeling dominated and controlled by others.

The exploration of a rupture in the alliance can lead to an in-depth exploration of a vicious cycle that is being enacted in the here-and-now of the therapeutic relationship that may to varying degrees be related to the type of vicious cycles that are problematic for the patient in his or her everyday experience. During this type of exploration, it is critical for the therapist to work collaboratively with the patient to explore the current transaction in its own terms and not to make any assumptions about the extent to which the current interaction reflects relational patterns that are characteristic for the patient. As we will discuss later, this type of open-ended exploration is consistent with the type of two-person psychology that underlies contemporary relational thinking and that is central to our approach.

Exploring core relational themes underlying alliance ruptures constitutes the central focus of this manual. In exploring such themes, it is critical for therapists to explore their own contribution to the interaction. For example, a therapist may contribute to his patient's feelings of being sexually exploited by deriving voyeuristic pleasure from hearing his patient discuss her sexual feelings and fantasies. A patient who has a readiness to feel intruded upon may be particularly reticent, thereby evoking an intrusive response in the frustrated therapist.

> Shelly was a 44-year-old woman who had been married for 20 years and had three children. She began treatment approximately 6 months after starting an affair with a married man. When she began treatment, any feelings of guilt or concerns about her marriage were of secondary importance to her. She was more immediately concerned that she was prone to experiencing intense pangs of jealousy whenever her lover showed any interest in other women. It emerged that Shelly had experienced similar feelings of jealousy in relation to her husband at the beginning of their marriage. These feelings had, however, disappeared long ago, and the marriage had been emotionally dead and passionless for many years. What was particularly striking to the therapist was the type of vague, gray, and washed-out quality to Shelly's presentation and the apparent lack of texture or any kind of emotional richness to her inner world. Queries about her inner experience or the mean-

ing of events to her were typically met with uninformative, one-sentence answers, and requests for elaboration were no more successful. Over time the therapist became increasingly aware of the way in which Shelly's reticence led him to intensify his efforts to extract material from her or to force his way into her inner world, and he began to explicitly examine the nature of their interaction with her. "It feels to me like I'm trying to force things out of you," he said, "and my guess is that it doesn't feel very good to you." This initiated a process of exploration that gradually began to illuminate different aspects of a core relational theme for Shelly.

She was able to begin articulating a fundamental belief that others would never be able to deeply value or cherish her. This belief made it difficult for her to value her own experience and robbed her of the ability to experience her inner world as meaningful, vivid, and alive. Shelly experienced the therapist's ongoing probing as a demand to perform, and came to feel increasingly inadequate and blocked by the pressure. She also spoke about a belief that any apparent interest in her by others (including the therapist) was transient or untrustworthy. For this reason, she felt a need to always hold part of herself back, so that, in her words, "There's some of myself I can save, even if I'm betrayed." Although at first she had difficulty acknowledging it, she subsequently began to become aware of feelings of resentment at the therapist for pressuring her. Later in treatment, her initially diminished concern for her husband and her marriage became more understandable in terms of similar buried feelings of resentment.

Indirect Focus on Tasks and Goals

Reframing the Meaning of Tasks and Goals. Reframing the meaning of therapeutic tasks and goals in terms that are acceptable to the patient is a type of joining intervention commonly used by strategic and systemic approaches (e.g., Minuchin & Fishman, 1981). For example, a patient who was receiving a cognitive-behavioral treatment for social anxiety was initially reluctant to complete any between-session assignments that involved increasing social contact because of a fear of rejection. When the therapist reframed the meaning of the assignment as one of "putting yourself into the anxiety-provoking situation in order to self-monitor your cognitive processes," the task no longer felt as risky, and she was willing to attempt the assignment. A patient in psychoanalytic treatment experienced his therapist's attempt to analyze his defenses as judgmental and unaccepting. When the therapist was able to frame the goal as one of increasing self-awareness and self-acceptance, rather than one of change, the alliance improved. It is critical for this type of intervention not to be delivered in a manipulative fashion. This requires that the therapist be able to genuinely view the reframe as a valid way of construing things, rather than as a white lie.

Changing Tasks and Goals. In this type of intervention, the therapist attempts to work on tasks and goals that seem relevant to the patient, rather than exploring factors underlying disagreements about tasks and goals. Whether or not the therapist and patient explicitly negotiate what the tasks and goals of therapy will consist of, there is always an implicit negotiation about how the patient's problems will be viewed and worked on. The therapist's ability and willingness to accommodate the patient by working in terms that are more meaningful to him or her can play a critical role not only in building the alliance in the immediate context, but also in helping the patient to develop a more generalized trust in the possibility of getting his or her own needs met in relationships with others. In some situations the decision to switch to a task that is more meaningful to the patient subsequently leads to a willingness on the patient's part to engage in other tasks that are initially viewed as more meaningful by the therapist. For example, treating a patient's phobia at a symptomatic level may help the patient develop sufficient trust to engage in the task of self-exploration later on. Accepting that it is difficult for a patient to explore her feelings and reducing the frequency of feeling-oriented questions may help her to feel sufficiently safe to explore her feelings at some later point.

Problems Associated with the Relational Bond

Direct Focus on the Relational Bond

Clarifying Misunderstandings. When the alliance becomes strained because the patient mistrusts the therapist or does not feel respected by the therapist, the therapist can attempt to clarify what is going on in the therapeutic interaction with an eye toward resolving misunderstandings, without actually addressing relational themes that are more core in nature. For example, a therapist who notices that her patient seems withdrawn initiates an exploration of what is going on in the here-and-now of the therapeutic relationship. The patient acknowledges that he feels hurt by something the therapist has said. The therapist then proceeds to explore the nature of the misunderstanding.

In this type of exploration, it can be critical for therapists to acknowledge their contribution to the misunderstanding. For example, the therapist becomes aware of the fact that she had indeed been somewhat critical in her remarks and acknowledges this to the patient. With this type of alliance-building intervention, the emphasis is on repairing a temporary strain in the alliance in order to permit the negotiation of other therapeutic tasks. For example, the therapist and patient may work through a temporary misunderstanding and then proceed to explore the patient's feeling about an event that took place outside of therapy. Nevertheless, the simple process of being able to talk about the misunderstanding and to experience the therapist responding in an empathic and nondefensive way can constitute an important new experience for the patient in the constructive negotiation of misunderstandings.

Exploring Core Relational Themes. Just as the exploration of disagreements about task and goals can lead to the exploration of important underlying themes, the exploration of strains in the bond aspect of the alliance, or of factors making it difficult to develop a bond in the first place, can ultimately lead to a working through of core relational themes. For example, a patient's feeling of being misattuned to by his therapist may lead to the exploration of a characteristic relational experience of being misunderstood by others. A feeling of being patronized by the therapist may lead to the exploration of a characteristic relational theme of being patronized by others. In this type of exploration, the resolution of a strain in the alliance becomes the therapeutic task rather than a necessary precondition for the successful completion of other therapeutic tasks. In some cases, the greater part of the treatment can focus on this type of therapeutic task. This is particularly likely to be the case with patients who begin treatment with a fundamental level of mistrust or skepticism about the value of therapy.

> Andrew was a graduate student in clinical psychology who began treatment, in part, because his training program strongly recommended that students acquire some experience as patients in treatment while completing their graduate training. From the outset, it was clear that he was extremely ambivalent about being in treatment and skeptical regarding its potential benefits. He had spent 4 years in treatment with a previous therapist as an undergraduate and had found it to be of little value. Over time the exploration of his skepticism helped him to articulate his belief that it was highly unlikely that anybody could teach him anything or help him learn something about himself that he didn't already know. His father had died when he was 10 years old, and his mother had been depressed and emotionally withdrawn. There had been a role reversal in his relationship with his mother, and in some respects he had acted as her therapist. He had developed a precocious maturity and had learned to play the role of the therapist with his friends at an early age. Over time it emerged in treatment that he

had a narcissistic investment in seeing himself as the "wise one" and that he experienced the role of the patient as degrading and intrinsically injurious to his self-esteem. On the one hand, he had an investment in viewing the therapist as incapable of helping him learn something new about himself. On the other hand, he had a desperate yearning to have somebody play the role of the mentor who could provide him with the type of guidance he had not received as an adolescent and a young man.

Psychoanalytically oriented treatments, with their emphasis on the exploration of transference–countertransference matrices, are more likely to focus on this level than other modalities. Is it conceptually problematic to equate the exploration of the transference with the working through of core themes that emerge out of the exploration of strains in the bond aspect of the alliance? In some respects, it is conceptually cleaner to maintain a distinction between alliance and transference and to view the alliance as the precondition that makes the exploration of the transference possible. This avoids the conceptual difficulty of having to maintain that development of an alliance is both a precondition for therapeutic tasks and an important task in its own right. It also avoids the difficulty raised by the question of whether some type of alliance is necessary in order to work on the alliance. On the other hand, we have already considered the problems with making a clear distinction between the alliance and transference. The assumption that the alliance is reasonable and the transference is irrational buys into an overly rationalistic model of the therapeutic process and raises the question of who (the therapist or the patient) is in the position to decide what is rational and what is irrational.

An alternative to this bind can be found in a multiple selves perspective (e.g., Bromberg, 1996; Mitchell, 1992; see Chapter 2), which holds that there is no unitary self split along the lines of rational versus irrational or conscious versus unconscious, but rather multiple selves that are always competing with one another for dominance. Although the tension between rational versus irrational self-states may come into play at different points during the exploration of strains in the therapeutic bond, other dimensions are relevant as well. For example, there may be an aspect of the self that feels more trusting and one that feels less trusting. Or there may be an aspect of the self that feels hopeful and one that is despairing. Trust or hope may have little to do with rationality. In fact, given a history of traumatic experiences, aspects of the self that are more trusting and hopeful may be quite irrational.

In order to directly work on core relational themes that emerge out of the exploration of strains in the bond aspect of the alliance, it is necessary for patients to have some access to the more trusting and hopeful aspects of their self-experience at the same time as they explore their more mistrusting and despairing self-states. Sometimes this can be facilitated by reiterating the rationale for this type of therapeutic task and obtaining the patient's explicit agreement to engage in this type of exploration. In situations when it is more difficult, however, it may be necessary to work on problems in the bond aspect of the alliance in a more indirect fashion.

Indirect Focus on the Relational Bond

Allying with the Resistance. One common form of allying with the resistance involves framing the patient's defensive avoidance of painful feelings as adaptive.

> Jennifer was a 38-year-old single woman who sought treatment in part because of her difficulty establishing a long-term romantic relationship with a man. As she approached her 40s, the pressure to have a child before her childbearing years were over intensified, along with her fear of never finding a mate. In treatment, a central issue that emerged was her fear of abandonment and her resulting difficulty in sharing feelings of need with other people and letting them in. In one session she began to explore her feelings of isolation and fear of spending the rest of her life alone in a particularly poignant fashion, and for the first time in treatment began to cry. She then became self-conscious, remarking that she was being melodramatic, and proceeded to talk about her situation in a more distant, intellectualized fashion. The therapist asked her to turn her attention inward for a moment.

THERAPIST (T): Just be aware for a moment of whether you're in contact with your pain or more distant from it right now.

JENNIFER (J): I'm more distant.

T: Uh huh . . . so that's okay and perhaps it's adaptive for you to have some distance from it right now.

J: Uh huh.

T: You know . . . maybe you need . . .

J: I have to go out into the street.

T: Yeah . . . so maybe you need some distance.

J: Uh huh.

T: As long as you're able to be aware of the way in which your talking about it helps you to distance from that immediate experience of a few moments back . . .

J: Yeah, thank God.

T: It's hard to stay in that place?

J: Yeah . . . staying in that place is so painful . . . (*She starts to cry again.*)

T: You start to contact the feelings again . . . (*Jennifer continues to cry.*)

This brief example illustrates the way in which allying with the resistance rather than challenging it can help patients to access avoided aspects of experience.

A second form of allying with the resistance involves validating mistrusting and despairing aspects of the self. In situations where patients have difficulty accessing more trusting and hopeful parts of the self, therapists may find it useful to spend considerable time allying with the more mistrusting and despairing aspects of the self. This process can gradually transform the situation so that patients can ultimately bring the more hopeful aspects of the self into the treatment. For example, a patient despaired about the possibility of being helped by the therapist, maintaining that he did not feel trusting enough to talk about important and embarrassing concerns. The therapist responded that it was appropriate for the patient not to trust her since she had not yet earned his trust. She thus empathized with the underlying mistrust. Furthermore, she maintained that for the patient to experience his mistrust in the context of the therapeutic relationship right now was "the work of therapy" and that there was nothing that he should be doing other than what he was doing.

New Relational Experience. A final intervention involves addressing the bond component of the alliance through actions, rather than through direct exploration. By refraining from acting in a way that confirms the patient's maladaptive relational schema or by unhooking from a vicious cycle that is being enacted, therapists can provide patients with a new relational experience that will help them to modify existing schemas. This type of intervention is particularly important when the patient has difficulty explicitly exploring the therapeutic relationship in the here-and-now. For example, the narcissistic patient who experiences an attempt to explore the therapeutic relationship as an impingement may need to be responded to with a holding environment (Winnicott, 1965) in which the therapist struggles to remain emotionally available to the patient while temporarily dealing with whatever complex and ambivalent feelings are aroused within at a private level (Slochower, 1997). Wilfred Bion's (1962) notion of *containment* (i.e., processing whatever distressing feelings are aroused in the therapist in a nondefensive fashion) is also relevant here. Thomas Ogden's (1994) concept of *interpretive action* provides another interesting perspective on this type of intervention. According to him, the therapist can communicate his understanding of what is going on through action, rather than through words. For example, a therapist decides to answer a patient's request for advice because he formulates the situation as one in which his decision to do so will position him in contrast to her abandoning father. A therapist decides not to lower her fees in response to the patient's request because she hypothesizes that the patient will experience himself as having conned the therapist.

> Ashley, a single young woman, working in an advertising firm, began treatment because of a general sense of emptiness and meaninglessness in her life. When she first started treatment, the therapist was struck by an interesting combination of emotional reserve and cautiousness, alternating with periodic eruptions of intense sadness which was surprisingly close to the surface. He was also struck by her caustic wit, a kind of a gallows humor. Ashley had grown up in a highly dysfunctional family. Her father was a hypercritical, sadistic man, who beat the children with minimal provocation and cheated on his wife regularly. Her mother was a chronically unhappy woman who consoled herself with alcohol and developed a serious drinking problem. Both parents neglected the emotional and physical needs of the six children in the family, who in many ways were left to raise themselves.
>
> On one occasion Ashley told the therapist a story about a shared experience with a friend of hers in high school that had been very meaningful to her. Her friend had a similar background of neglect and abuse, and she and Ashley had felt a mutual kinship early in their acquaintance. Once a teacher in class had told them about Harry Harlow's classic experiments with monkeys and surrogate mothers, and the two girls had found the image of the young monkeys clinging to the surrogate mother for contact comfort hysterically funny. Ashley was not able to explain to the therapist why this image had seemed so funny to her, but it struck him as a poignant metaphorical encapsulation of the pain and emotional deprivation she had experienced in her life.
>
> In the early phases of treatment, Ashley had considerable difficulty exploring painful topics and feelings, and any attempt to explore what was taking place in the therapeutic relationship was rejected as pointless and irrelevant. She began most sessions with superficial chit-chat and then lapsed into an angry silence, as if waiting for the therapist to do something for her. Ashley spent

considerable time talking about the fact that she wasn't finding therapy helpful and was considering leaving. When the therapist asked her what was missing, she replied that she needed more guidance and direction. She also reported feeling uncomfortable and mistrusting because of the therapist's relative lack of self-disclosiveness. The therapist spent some time attempting to explore what these concerns meant to her and how she experienced his current stance, but was unable to make much progress. Ashley questioned the value of this line of inquiry and maintained that she didn't know what his questions really meant. She felt that he was "playing the role of therapist."

Without fully understanding the meaning or Ashley's request for more guidance, but having a semiarticulated formulation regarding the importance for her of receiving the kind of guidance and support she had never experienced as a child, the therapist began to experiment with being more active and providing advice about the various dilemmas she would raise. For example, on one occasion Ashley asked his opinion about how to handle a fight with her boyfriend, and the therapist suggested a strategy. He also began to experiment with being more self-disclosive, hypothesizing that she was experiencing his reserve as withholding and abandoning. It was as if Ashley's request for more self-disclosure on the therapist's part was a way of saying, "I'm not going to take the risk of opening up in this relationship until you prove that you're willing to invest in it by taking emotional risks." So, for example, when Ashley asked the therapist whether he ever felt that things were meaningless or had doubts about the vocational path he had chosen (both concerns for her), he would provide brief but genuine answers. At the same time, he monitored her responses closely. He noted that responses of this type seemed to free her up to talk more openly about herself. He also noted that she seemed careful not to push the boundary too far by asking questions that he experienced as overly demanding or intrusive. Over time, the tension started to ease between them, and Ashley began to move in the direction of greater trust and openness.

※ 2

Fundamental Assumptions
and Principles

In this chapter, we outline a number of general assumptions and principles that provide a useful foundation for working through ruptures in the therapeutic alliance. This is not intended as a systematic theoretical framework, but rather as an attempt to highlight critical issues and themes. These principles are of a more general nature and are relevant to the way that therapists orient themselves toward psychotherapy as a whole. At the same time, they have important implications for the way in which we view the clinical process during therapeutic impasses. For example, the assumption that agency and relatedness are fundamental human needs in human beings, and the related assumptions that they are in ongoing tension with one another, provide a useful framework for understanding the types of conflicts that underlie many ruptures in the therapeutic alliance. A constructivist epistemology is more consistent with a stance of genuine openness and humility on the therapist's part (which from our perspective is critical in the context of an alliance rupture) than a realist epistemology is. A two-person psychology (i.e., the view that both therapist and patient are always contributing to the character of the patient–therapist interaction) is more consistent with a stance in which the therapist tries to understand his or her own contribution to what is taking place than a one-person psychology is (i.e., the view that the therapist can be a neutral observer who stands outside the interaction). Contemporary emotion theory and research can shed light on the complex role that affective commu-

30

nication between patients and therapists can play in therapeutic impasses, as well as the role that therapists' emotions can play in discovering the route through those impasses.

AGENCY VERSUS RELATEDNESS

A number of different theoretical developments converge on the notion that human beings have innate needs both for establishing and maintaining relatedness with others and for self-definition or individuation (e.g., Bakan, 1966; Buber, 1936). These two needs are in conflict and exist in dialectical relation to one another. Otto Rank (1929, 1945) maintained that the process of maturation involves individuating from one's parents, and that this process inevitably produces guilt because it threatens relatedness to them. According to Michael Balint (1968), people are born into a natural state of "object relatedness." They tend to react to disturbances in this natural state in two general patterns: ocnophilic and philobatic. The *ocnophile* clings to the object in a dependent fashion and experiences intense anxiety when separation is threatened. The *philobat* attempts to protect himself from the threat of disruption of relatedness by shunning relationships and becoming excessively dependent on himself.

D. W. Winnicott (1965) believed that human beings have a fundamental need both for symbiosis with the other and for solitude. Margaret Mahler (1968) maintained that the infant has a desire both for symbiotic union with the mother and a natural tendency to individuate. Sidney Blatt (e.g., Blatt & Blass, 1992), in a manner that is reminiscent of Balint, distinguishes between two types of depression: anaclitic and introjective. *Anaclitic* depressives are anxiously dependent upon others, while *introjective* depressives are compulsively self-reliant and preoccupied with the struggle for self-definition.

Jay Greenberg (1991), in his attempt to reformulate Freud's dual instinct theory, replaces libido and aggression with effectance and security. *Effectance* consists of the drive to establish one's sense of agency, while *security* consists of the drive for interpersonal relatedness. Greenberg suggests that intrapsychic conflict can be understood in terms of the conflicting needs for effectance and security. More recently, Lewis Aron (1996), in his comprehensive review and synthesis of contemporary relational theory, delineates these two conflicting needs as fundamental to human nature and argues that they must be balanced in our conceptualization of the therapeutic process.

Interestingly, these two dimensions also underlie all interpersonal circumplex conceptualizations of personality (e.g., Plutchik & Conte, 1997). These models assume that

> all human interpersonal behavior represents blends of two basic motivations: the need for control (power, dominance) and the need for affiliation (love, friendliness). Persons interacting with each other continually negotiate two major personality issues: how friendly or hostile they will be with each other, and how much in charge or in control each will be in their encounters. (Kiesler, 1996, pp. 7–8)

This two-dimensional conceptualization of the fundamental nature of human experience has important implications for understanding both normal and abnormal development. On the one hand, the needs for agency and relatedness are in conflict with one another. As Rank (1929, 1945) suggested, the process of individuating is inherently guilt-producing and fraught with anxiety since it threatens relatedness. Paradoxically, the attainment of true individuation and relatedness are dependent upon one another. As theorists such as Mahler (1968) and John Bowlby (1988) have suggested, the infant requires a sense of security in relationship with the caretaker before she can engage in the type of exploratory behavior necessary to facilitate individuation. Conversely, one cannot maintain a mature form of relatedness to others until one has developed a sense of oneself as an individual.

The resolution of the tension between the need for agency and the need for relatedness is a dialectic that lies at the heart of psychoanalytic theory. The classical position on this issue is that the patient expresses infantile needs and impulses that are inappropriate to the current situation. The therapist's job is to allow these needs and impulses to emerge in the form of the transference, which is then analyzed; the therapist's role is to understand rather than to gratify these needs and impulses. From this perspective, primary process ultimately is changed through secondary process. Patients acknowledge their infantile needs and desires and then tame or modulate them (Eagle, 1984).

From the early days of psychoanalytic theory, however, there were dissenters to this position. Wilhelm Reich (1949), for example, came to see the free expression of libidinal energy as the ultimate therapeutic goal. Reich's worldview is a romantic one that idealizes man's natural instinct. This position is a thread carried through a number of more contemporary positions. For example, Fritz Perls (1973), who was analyzed by Reich, argued that the spontaneous expression of emotion is a major goal of psychotherapy. This became a central theme in the humanistic psychotherapies. An important assumption in these traditions is that there is a self-actualizing tendency and that people who return to their natural state will automatically find a harmonious way of living with others.

Another alternative to the classical perspective can be traced back to Rank (1945) and his emphasis on the importance of the will in healthy functioning and in therapeutic change (see Chapter 3). This perspective recognizes the inherent tension between agency and relatedness. Rank saw the paralysis of the will, which results from the attempt to accommodate others, as the source of psychopathology.

Yet another alternative to the clinical classical position on this issue can be traced back to Ferenczi (1933). Ferenczi argued that children are traumatized by the empathic failures of their parents, and that they split off part of themselves in order to relate to others. He also argued that ultimately the trauma that the patient experienced as a child would be reenacted in the context of the current therapeutic relationship and that this reenactment would allow the patient to work through the conflicts with the therapist in a new way which did not involve disowning parts of the self.

As we will see in Chapter 3, this theme subsequently emerges in different forms in the work of theorists such as Balint, Winnicott, and Kohut. In this alternative to classical theory, the solution to the fundamental conflict lies neither in the renunciation of infantile impulses nor in their free expression. Instead, it involves a maturational process emerging out of the negotiation between the needs of self and other. This alternative involves the paradoxical acceptance of both the validity of one's needs and the reality of the fact that they will not always be satisfied, a theme we shall return to later.

In what has become a cornerstone for the relational perspective in psychoanalysis, Stephen Mitchell (1988) contrasted Freud's view of the change process with a contemporary relational perspective. He argued that while Freud believed that change takes place through renunciation of instinctual needs and the development of rational understanding, relational theory emphasizes the development of a richer, more authentic sense of self.

In contemporary culture, more than ever before, high value is placed upon individuation. In more traditional societies, the idea of one's relationship to oneself or the existential ethic of authenticity had no real meaning. The fundamental moral question was not how one related to one's inner self, but rather how one related to some universal set of ethical principles. With the downfall of such a set of principles, and the development of a more individuated self, the question of how one relates to oneself becomes more meaningful.

Freud's emphasis on the conflict between instinct and civilization can be understood as a particular cultural expression of the underlying tension between the needs for agency versus the needs for relatedness. In contemporary culture this tension takes a different form. With the progressive development of the individuated self and the breakdown of shared cultural values and prescribed role relationships, it has become increasingly important for individuals to develop their own personal sense of meaning and to find ways of feeling connected to others in the context of an increasingly fragmented society.

We thus agree with Mitchell that the development of a richer, more authentic sense of self constitutes an important therapeutic goal. It is important, however, to recognize that this emphasis on the development of the self reflects contemporary cultural developments that value the "masterful, bounded self" (Cushman, 1995) at the expense of the more communal aspects of human existence. Conceptualizing the therapeutic goal as one of developing a richer, more authentic self in some respects perpetuates some of the imbalances of the excessively individualistic culture, which has given rise to some of the current shifts in psychotherapy theory. Conceptualizing the goal of treatment as learning to constructively negotiate the need for agency versus the need for relatedness thus provides a broader, more comprehensive framework for change than the goal of self-development. This perspective is very much compatible with a view of therapy as a process of intersubjective negotiation (e.g., Aron, 1996; Mitchell, 1993; Pizer, 1992). And, as we shall discuss subsequently, it provides a useful metatheoretical framework for viewing the processes through which ruptures in the therapeutic alliance are negotiated.

CONSTRUCTIVISM AND REALISM

The shift toward constructivism cuts across diverse therapeutic orientations, including the psychoanalytic (e.g., Hoffman, 1994; Stern, 1997), the cognitive (e.g., Guidano, 1987; Mahoney, 1991), the experiential (e.g., Gendlin, 1994; Greenberg et al., 1993), and the systemic/strategic (e.g., Coyne & Pepper, 1998; Watzlawick, 1978), and is consistent with a more general cultural shift toward a postmodern sensibility. This shift has a number of important therapeutic implications. One of the most important is that it challenges the traditional view that the therapist can have some privileged understanding of reality, whether that reality is the patient's internal reality (as in classical psychoanalysis) or external reality (as in rationalist cognitive therapy). It is thus consistent with a more egalitarian view of the therapeutic relationship. This type of shift can be extremely important in helping therapists to work through therapeutic impasses in which the inherent power imbalance in the therapeutic relationship can perpetuate the problem and play a role in blinding the therapist to the validity of the patient's perspective.

The position espoused in this book is not a radical constructivism, but rather what Irwin Hoffman (1998) has referred to as a "dialectical constructivism." This is a position that navigates a middle road between the extremes of nihilism, on the one hand, and naive realism, on the other. The task of finding this middle road is a central preoccupation for many contemporary philosophers of science (e.g., Bernstein, 1983; Habermas, 1987).

Hans-Georg Gadamer's (1960) hermeneutic perspective provides a resolution of the dilemma that is particularly congenial to us (see also Stern, 1997). He argues that one's perception of reality is always constrained by one's preconceptions or prejudices. These preconceptions are, however, more than just a limiting factor. They also function as the ground for all experience, since without preconceptions new experience is meaningless. The task, nevertheless, remains one of finding some way of moving beyond our preconceptions so that we are able to move toward apprehending the "thing itself." Gadamer argues that it is possible to take this step and thus move beyond solipsism, and that there are two necessary aspects to this process. The first involves becoming aware of our preconceptions and the way in which they currently shape our understanding. The second involves testing our preconceptions through open dialogue or "genuine conversation." This dialogue can take place in relationship to other human beings or to something else (e.g., textual interpretation). In both cases, however, one has to be truly open to changing one's perception in response to an adequate challenge. Central to Gadamer's thinking is the notion that dialogue of this type not only allows two people to come to an understanding of one another's positions, but also allows them to arrive at a better understanding of things as they really are. Thus, although there is no ideal reality independent of the perceiver, reality is more than simply a reflection of the perceiver's mind. In a sense, then, truth is *both* constructed *and* discovered.

As Buddhist philosophers of the Centrist school have maintained since the second century C.E., it is critical to recognize that the idea of constructivism is itself a construct. It has no more inherent reality than the position of naive realism. The notion of constructivism can best be thought of as a corrective to the stance of naive realism, in other words, as a medicine for the disease of naive realism. Like any medicine, too much of it can make one ill. Radical constructivism and naive realism are thus both epistemological errors; as Buddhist philosophy observes, of the two errors, nihilism is the more dangerous (Williams, 1989).

BEGINNER'S MIND: THE DANGERS OF REIFICATION

Given the way in which preconceptions can limit our ability to see what is taking place, it is critical for therapists to learn to become aware of and then to let go of their preconceptions as they emerge. Wilfred Bion's (1967) oft-quoted and controversial advice that therapists should approach every session "without memory and desire" was an important attempt to convey the value of this type of mental discipline for the therapist. The Zen master Shunru Suzuki (1970) spoke about this discipline as one of cultivating a *beginner's mind*. In his words, "If your mind is empty, it is always ready for anything; it is open to everything. In the beginner's mind, there are many possibilities; in the expert's mind, there are few" (p. 21). In the Buddhist tradition of mindfulness meditation, this has been otherwise referred to as "disciplined not knowing" and "bare attention" (see Epstein, 1995).

Ernst Schactel (1959) has described a similar attitude with his notion of *allocentricity,* which entails a curiosity, an openness or receptivity, that requires the tolerance of ambiguity, uncertainty, and sometimes pain as well. It involves a profound interest in the whole object, a full turning toward the object, which makes possible a direct encounter with it (not merely a quick registration of its familiar features according to ready labels). To approach another as such is to be as curious as possible, open to all the alternate formulations one finds unfinished in oneself, including one's reactions to the other. And finally, Martin Buber (1923) spoke eloquently about the importance of being able to treat every moment as a new moment and to be open to what it has to reveal in its fullness and in all of its particularities.

> In spite of all similarities every living situation has, like a newborn child, a new face that has never been before and will never come again. It demands of you a reaction which cannot be prepared beforehand. It demands nothing of what is past. It demands presence, responsibility; it demands you. I call a great character one who by his actions and attitudes satisfies the claim of situations out of deep readiness to respond with his whole life, and in such a way that the sum of his actions and attitudes expresses at the same time the unity of his being in its willingness to accept responsibility. (Buber, 1923, p. 114)

Therapy is an ongoing flow of moments that are woven together through a process of construction. While this construction is a useful and necessary part of making sense of what is going on in psychotherapy, it can also stand in the way of approaching things at a level that is sufficiently subtle to allow therapists to see new openings for intervention as they emerge. It is important to remember that new information and new possibilities are constantly emerging in every moment of interaction with the patient. The therapist who is able to let go of his or her current understanding of what is happening in order to see what is emerging in the moment will have more flexibility and adaptability to the situation than the therapist who cannot do so.

One is always going to have preconceptions that shape one's perception of the current situation, and one is always going to have theories that shape one's stance toward the patient. To suggest that the therapist abandon such theories and preconceptions completely would thus be unrealistic. Through a process of becoming aware of one's preconceptions in action, however, one can become more open to seeing things more fully. A primary factor standing in the way of approaching the situation with a *beginner's mind* is that it can be very anxiety-provoking to do psychotherapy without the solid ground provided by the concepts one normally uses to impose order on what is going on. This anxiety can become particularly pronounced when one is caught in a therapeutic impasse that challenges one's sense of worth as a therapist.

Reification, or the failure to distinguish between one's constructs and the underlying phenomenon that these constructs represent, is one of the key sources of dysfunction in everyday life and one of the major roadblocks for therapists. As therapists, we must constantly struggle with the temptation to hold on to fixed conceptions of what is taking place between us and our patients. We must constantly struggle with the temptation to deal with the anxiety and discomfort of ambiguous situations and to establish some sense of security in the midst of the experience of groundlessness, through reification. Patients come to us for help, and our sense of competency and self-worth is based upon our ability to make sense of complex and confusing situations and to extract some sense of order and structure out of ambiguity and meaninglessness.

This is particularly true for new therapists who are struggling to gain an initial sense of competency, and whose sense of self-worth feels on the line in every moment. The same temptations, however, are present for more advanced therapists. One source of this temptation stems from the fact that more experienced therapists often feel that it is more difficult for them to acknowledge that they don't have the answers. Also, the more practiced and experienced they become, the easier it is for them to fall into habitual and routinized ways of looking at things. It is also tempting for therapists to grasp premature explanations of what is taking place in order to avoid looking at potentially threatening possibilities regarding the nature of their own contributions to interactions with their patients.

Reification takes many forms. At the more molar level are such forms of reification as seeing patients as examples of particular diagnostic labels or personality disorders. For example, relating to our patients as borderline or narcissistic, rather than as particular and unique individuals, is a manifestation of reification. A construct of this type can be useful in that it summarizes certain regularities in patterns that have been observed over time. It can thus be a valuable heuristic. At the same time, however, it can prevent therapists from seeing the underlying reality of the patient who is sitting in front of them and the unique interaction they are engaged in with their patient in any given moment.

A more molecular form of reification takes place when we make an inference about something, such as the patient's feelings or internal state, and then have difficulty seeing this inference as nothing more than a tentative hypothesis. For example, we believe that the patient is angry and have difficulty letting go of this perception, despite consistent denials on the patient's part.

A final form of reification takes place when we assume that something that was true about the patient or our interaction with the patient at one point in time is true at a second point in time. For example, a therapist in supervision became aware of a pattern in which his patient responded to confrontations with compliance. In the next session, he proceeded to comment on this pattern to his patient, who responded by denying it. The therapist persisted in confronting the patient with his compliance, without any awareness that a new relational configuration was emerging involving a power struggle between the two of them.

ONE-PERSON AND TWO-PERSON PSYCHOLOGIES

Much has been written in psychoanalytic theory on the distinction between one- and two-person psychologies (e.g., Aron, 1996; Balint, 1968; Ghent, 1989; Mitchell, 1988). Typically, theories greatly influenced by classical analysis have been cast as one-person psychologies, where the emphasis is on the individual experience of the patient, and the therapist is seen as a blank screen onto which the patient's fantasies are projected. The two-person psychological perspective has emerged in reaction to what its proponents view as the limitations of a one-person psychology. The American interpersonal tradition has been particularly influential in the development of a two-person psychology (although it was Michael Balint, 1968, who coined the term).

In a two-person psychology, the patient–therapist relationship is the object of study, and the therapist is considered a coparticipant, rather than one who can stand outside of the interpersonal field and observe. The fundamental premise is, to quote Harry Stack Sullivan (1954), that the therapist "has an inescapable, inextricable involvement in all that goes on in the interview; and to the extent that he is unconscious or unwitting of his participation in the interview, to that extent he does not know what is happening" (p. 19). The therapist can never be an impartial observer who stands apart from the phenomenon being observed. Jay Greenberg (1995) captures this sense of coparticipation or mutuality with his concept of the *interactive matrix*. According to him,

> The interactive matrix is shaped, from moment to moment in every treatment, by the personal characteristics of the analysand and of the analyst. These include the beliefs, commitments, hopes, fears, needs, and wishes of both participants. It is only within the context of the interactive matrix that the events of an analysis acquire their meaning. (p. 1)

From this perspective, countertransference becomes the normal state of affairs rather than an episodic phenomenon, and the therapist who thinks he understands the nature of his participation in a definitive fashion is in trouble.

The two-person perspective has a number of important clinical implications. First, it suggests that clinical formulations must always be guided by and revised in light of information gleaned from an ongoing exploration of what is taking place in the here-and-now of the therapeutic relationship. Second, it is critical for the therapist to engage in an ongoing exploration of his or her contributions to the interaction. Third, it is never safe to assume that the interaction emerging in the therapy session parallels patterns that are characteristic of the patient's daily life. The extent to which the relationship between the therapist and the patient parallels other relationships in the patient's life must always be kept an open question.

As the field has come to recognize the importance of a two-person perspective, it has changed the conceptualization of the nature of the therapeutic relationship. As described earlier, in classical psychoanalytic theory a distinction was made between those patient feelings toward the therapist that are reality-based and those that are transferential in nature. From a constructivist perspective, this distinction is difficult to maintain, since it implies that the therapist is in the privileged position of being able to judge what is real and what is not real. It cannot be assumed that the patient's relationship to the therapist is more transferential in nature than the therapist's relationship to the patient since all experience in the present is determined by previous experience. This perspective was anticipated in the humanistic/experiential tradition by theorists such as Carl Rogers (1951, 1957) who definitively rejected the concept of transference.

Many contemporary analysts are reluctant to make a clear-cut distinction between the therapeutic relationship and other relationships. Arnold Modell (1991), for example, argues that the therapeutic relationship is both real and unreal, and that it is the paradoxical nature of this relationship that allows for the possibility of change. To view the patient's feelings as nothing but transference can serve a defensive function for the therapist and invalidate the patient's experience. On the other hand, to treat the patient's feelings toward the therapist completely at face value, without inquiring into their complex, multi-determined nature, can be to miss a valuable opportunity for exploration.

Owen Renik (1998) goes a step further than Modell in emphasizing that far from being not quite real, the therapeutic relationship is "a *very real* relationship, no different in its reality from any other, taking place within the protective limits provided by the agreed-upon ground rules of the analytic contract" (p. 115). His point is that the special parameters of the therapeutic relationship (e.g., its asymmetry and the agreement not to meet outside of the scheduled time slot) do not make it unreal any more than the parameters of other relationships (e.g., teacher–student, doctor–patient) make them unreal.

There has also been a movement toward eliminating the distinction between those therapeutic feelings that are countertransferential and those that are not, since the ability to make such a distinction implies a type of objectivity precluded by a constructivist perspective. Moreover, the very term *countertransference* implies that the therapist's feelings are a reaction to the patient, rather than an equal component in an interaction that is mutual in nature (Wolstein, 1988).

As Aron (1996) suggests, it is important to recognize that there are different aspects to this mutuality. One aspect involves the process of mutual regulation between patient and therapist. Patient and therapist influence one another on an ongoing basis at both conscious and unconscious levels. A second involves the ongoing negotiation of tasks, goals, parameters, and even the basic substance of therapy. A third consists of the role that the authentic encounter between patient and therapist can play in the change process. It is also important to recognize that, as Aron maintains, mutuality does not necessarily imply symmetry. There is an inherent asymmetry in the roles of patient and therapist, and certain aspects of this asymmetry need to be maintained if the therapist is going to be helpful to the patient.

As Irwin Hoffman (1994) points out, society invests the therapist with a special kind of power, mystique, and authority that have a positive impact on the therapeutic process. Therapists cannot completely eliminate this aura, even if they want to, and to deny the presence of this aspect of the asymmetry entails a certain type of inauthenticity. Moreover, the various prescriptions associated with the therapist's role and the parameters of the treatment (e.g., not meeting with patients for coffee, being selective in terms of what one self-discloses) have other important therapeutic functions. For example, they can allow the patient to feel safe to explore themes that would be too risky to explore in other relationships. They can also help the therapists feel sufficiently safe to become aware of their own feelings and fantasies and harness them for the therapeutic process.

From Hoffman's perspective, the therapist's task is to strike a balance between acting in accordance with the role prescriptions of the therapist, on the one hand, and, on the other hand, acting in a fashion that is self-expressive and sufficiently spontaneous to allow a bond of mutual identification to develop. In fact, the asymmetrical nature of the therapeutic relationship makes our participation with our patients in the spirit of mutuality matter more to them than it would otherwise. According to Hoffman, impasses and traumatic treatments take place when therapists commit themselves to either side of this dialectic in an uncritical fashion. Conversely, it is the therapist's struggle to find the right balance between these two poles, in a fashion that is responsive to the needs of the unique interactive matrix that emerges with each patient, that is particularly therapeutic.

INTERVENTIONS AS RELATIONAL ACTS

In addition to whatever explicit informational value an intervention contains, it must also be understood as a relational act (Aron, 1996; Mitchell, 1988). In this regard, it is useful to make the distinction between the content and the process dimensions of communication. As communication theorists maintain (Watzlawick, Beavin, & Jackson, 1967), there are always report and command aspects to any communication. The *report* aspect of the communication is the explicit content of the communication. The *command* aspect of the communication is the implicit interpersonal statement that is being conveyed by the communication.

For example, the cognitive therapist who uses Socratic questioning to help the patient see a more adaptive viewpoint may be position-

ing himself as a teacher vis-à-vis a student and implying that he ultimately knows the answer toward which he is guiding the patient. The
person-centered therapist or self psychologist who emphasizes empathic reflections or experience-near interpretations may be conveying the
message that she is a midwife and that the patient is the final arbiter of
his own experience. The Kleinian analyst, who makes a deep interpretation of the patient's unconscious, may be taking the role of the one
who knows in relation to the patient who has no direct access to an aspect of her experience.

None of these relational statements are inherently good or bad. As is
always the case, good or bad depends upon the context. For example, the
therapist who positions himself as the one who knows may inspire hope
in a particular patient who is feeling hopeless and demoralized. But the
same stance might make another patient feel patronized. One patient
may feel respected by the therapist who restricts his interventions to
empathic reflections and inspired to feel trust in his own experience; another may feel frustrated or abandoned by the same intervention.

A therapist who interprets in a definitive fashion conveys a different
message about the relationship than one who interprets more tentatively.
In certain contexts, a definitively offered interpretation can be experienced as particularly helpful by the patient. It can reassure the patient
that the therapist has something substantial to offer him or her and that
the therapist is willing to act on his or her behalf. On the other hand, an
interpretation of this type can be experienced as accurate by the patient
without necessarily being helpful. As Rogers (1951) argued early on, and
as contemporary analysts are increasingly coming to recognize (e.g.,
Bollas, 1987; Winnicott, 1986), such an interpretation can deprive the patient of the vital experience of self-discovery. Moreover, a patient may accept an interpretation in order to maintain relatedness to the therapist. It
is thus critical for the therapist to monitor the relational implications of
his or her interventions on an ongoing basis. It is also critical for the therapist to monitor the motivation underlying his or her interpretations. Is
he making a definitive interpretation in order to affirm his own sense of
potency? Is the desire to feel potent fueled by the patient's interpersonal
stance? Is he reluctant to say anything definitive for fear of being criticized or rejected? Is this fear a consistent theme for him? Is it related to
some aspect of the patient's style?

MOTIVATION AND EMOTION

There is a movement afoot in diverse therapeutic traditions to develop
a comprehensive motivational theory grounded in contemporary emo-

tion theory and research (e.g., Greenberg & Safran, 1987; Jones, 1995; Lichtenberg, 1989; Safran & Greenberg, 1991; Spezzano, 1993; Westen, 1997). Central to this theory is the notion that emotions are biologically wired into the human organism through an evolutionary process and that they play an adaptive role in the survival of the species. Emotions function to safeguard the concerns of the organism (Ekman & Davidson, 1994; Frijda, 1986; Spezzano, 1993). Some of these concerns or goals (e.g., attachment) are biologically programmed, while others are learned. Emotions are conceptualized as a form of action disposition information. They provide us with internal feedback about the actions that we are prepared to engage in. They provide us with information about the self as a biological organism, with a particular history, in interaction with the environment. As such, they are at the core of subjective and intersubjective meaning (Spezzano, 1993).

It is useful to understand the structure underlying the fundamental sequences of social behavior in terms of motivational systems that have been wired into the human species through a process of natural selection. Examples include attachment, exploration, sexual excitement, flight, and aggression (e.g., Bowlby, 1988; Jones, 1995; Spezzano, 1993). Emotions function as the subjective readout (or experiential monitor) of which motivational systems or combinations of systems are dominant at any given time. These systems become activated in response to the appraisal (which is typically only partially conscious) of various environmental contingencies. For example, anger occurs in response to events experienced as an assault or violation. It informs the individual of his or her organismic preparedness to engage in aggressive behavior. Sadness occurs in response to a loss and organismically prepares one to recover or compensate for what is lost. Fear is evoked by events appraised as dangerous and informs individuals of an organismic preparedness for flight. Emotions can thus be thought of as a type of embodied knowledge.

Contemporary psychoanalytic theory is in transition regarding motivational theory. Many contemporary theorists reject drive metapsychology as excessively mechanistic and as incompatible with a psychology of meaning. Furthermore, they argue that drive theory fails to recognize that human beings are intrinsically interpersonal creatures. Many theories of a more relational cast substitute the need for human relatedness for the traditional drives of sexuality and aggression. They fail, however, to provide a comprehensive model of human motivation.

A number of critics have argued that in rejecting drive theory, relational theorists have discarded one of the most important insights of classical psychoanalysis: that intrapsychic conflict is a central feature of human experience. Some, such as Mitchell (1988), have argued that conflict still plays an important role in psychopathology, but that the conflict is between different relational configurations rather than between instinct and society. This accounts for some forms of conflict (e.g., the conflict between different acquired values), but it does not account for the type of conflict that drive theory was originally designed to capture (i.e., the conflict between instinctually based wishes and socially acquired values).

From the perspective of emotion theory, the type of conflict focused on by classical theory can still be dealt with. There are, however, two important necessary theoretical refinements. The first is that intrapsychic conflict is not viewed as consisting of a tension between biologically based needs and socially acquired values, but rather a tension between two different types of psycho-/biologically based needs. In human beings, it is difficult to find purely biologically based instincts (Mitchell, 1988). Even sexuality and aggression have socially conditioned meanings. Conversely, even socially acquired values can be traced back to the biologically based need for relatedness.

The second is that the range of potentially conflictual instincts needs to be extended beyond sexuality and aggression to the full range of motivational systems that are biologically programmed into the human species and that at times may come into conflict with the attachment system (e.g., Lichtenberg, 1989). Thus, for example, an individual may learn that joy, curiosity, pride, or sadness are threatening to relatedness and thus may learn to dissociate the relevant aspects of self-experience (Safran & Segal, 1990).

Healthy functioning involves the integration of affective information with higher level cognitive processing in order to act in a fashion that is grounded in organismically based need, but not bound by reflexive action (Greenberg & Safran, 1987; Leventhal, 1984; Safran & Greenberg, 1991). Thus, for example, an individual may be aware of his anger at someone, but deem it unwise to respond aggressively. Individuals who have difficulty accessing the full range of their emotional experience, however, will be deprived of important information. They may suppress or fail to mobilize a motivational system that may be adaptive in a specific context. For example, the individual who has difficulty experiencing anger may fail to mobilize adaptive aggression. The individual who has difficulty experiencing more vulnerable feelings may fail to fulfill healthy needs for nurturance. A second consequence of the process of dissociating emotional experience is that there may be an incongruence between one's actions and subjective experience. Since the activation of a motivational system is not dependent on the conscious experience of the associated emotion, it is not uncommon for people to have only partial awareness of the impact they have on others. Thus, for example, the individual who dissociates feelings of anger may nevertheless act aggressively and evoke aggression in response. This type of duplicitous communication (Kaiser, 1965) can play a major role in psychopathology and in the type of complex alliance ruptures that emerge in therapy.

AFFECTIVE APPRAISAL AND COMMUNICATION

From the early days of psychoanalytic theory there has been an interest in the phenomenon of unconscious appraisal and communication. Sandor Ferenczi (1915) initially described a phenomenon that he referred to as "the dialogues of the unconsciouses . . . where the unconscious of two people completely understand themselves and each other, without the remotest conception of this on the part of the consciousness of either" (p. 109). Freud, Ferenczi, and Anna Freud engaged in "thought-transference" experiments together (Hidas, 1993). Ferenczi believed that psychoanalytic work could be enhanced by using the analyst's free association to read the patient's unconscious (Stanton, 1990).

Theodore Reik (1948) wrote extensively about the unconscious processes through which opinions are formed. He maintained that unconscious appraisal processes contribute considerably more to our impression of others than do conscious perceptions.

> We remember details of another person's dress and peculiarities in his gestures, without recalling them; a number of minor points, an olfactory nuance; a sense of touch while shaking hands, too slightly observed; warmth, clamminess, roughness or smoothness of the skin; the manner in which he glances up or looks—of all this we are not consciously aware, and yet it influences our opinion. The minutest movements accompany every process of thought; muscular twitches in face or hands and movements of the eyes speak to us as well as words. (p. 135)

Paula Heimann (1950), too, emphasized the importance of the therapist's emotions and unconscious processes in understanding the patient. She maintained that the emotions aroused in the therapist are much nearer to the heart of the matter than reasoning, or to put it in other words, the therapist's unconscious perception of the patient's unconscious is more acute and in advance of his or her conscious conception of the situation. Many contemporary analysts (e.g., Gabbard, 1995; Ogden, 1979; Joseph, 1989; Davies, 1996) have argued that the mechanism through which such unconscious perception and communication takes place is *projective identification*. They believe that patients pressure therapists to act in accordance with projected aspects of themselves, and in so doing unconsciously communicate dissociated aspects of their own experience.

Contemporary emotion research and theory has the potential to shed additional light on the mechanisms through which unconscious appraisal and communication take place. First, with respect to unconscious perception, emotions provide us with a rapid and economical appraisal of what events and interpersonal interactions mean to us as biological organisms. They are a form of tacit, unarticulated meaning, in that they tell us what things mean to us in terms of the actions we are prepared to engage in. They summarize a complex array of information that is processed at an unconscious level and results in a rapid, condensed, but nevertheless sophisticated, appraisal (Greenberg & Safran, 1987; Safran & Greenberg, 1991). Thus, for example, a feeling of wariness evoked by another person may be based upon multiple cues that are unconsciously perceived, such as tone of voice, quality of eye contact, and posture.

The phenomenon of unconscious communication becomes less mysterious when we recognize the central role that emotion plays in human interactions. Different emotions are linked to different distinct expressive–motor behaviors. The most compelling empirical evidence at this point in time is for the link between facial expression and emotion, although other consistent links may also exist (e.g., Ekman, 1993). While there is considerable controversy among emotion theorists and researchers about the functional relationship between emotion and nonverbal expression (e.g., Is the subjective experience of emotion partially generated by facial feedback?), there is considerable agreement that the expressive–motor aspects of emotion, particularly facial expression, play an important role in interpersonal communication. This, of course, makes good sense from an evolutionary perspective, given the fact that communication and cooperation is essential to the survival of the species. While verbal communication enables individuals to engage in abstract, symbolic exchanges, it is considerably less rapid and economical than nonverbal communication. Moreover, it is vulnerable to dissimulation.

While emotion provides the individual with a monitor of his or her own action dispositions, the expressive–motor behaviors associated with it provide others with an ongoing readout of these same action dispositions. While this process of reading the other's affective displays can have a conscious element to it, a good deal of it takes place out of awareness, in the same way that other affective appraisals take place. Thus, for example, we may unconsciously appraise the other's aggressive disposition toward us, and in turn feel angry (i.e., be prepared to reciprocate with aggression), without being fully aware of either our own readiness to be aggressive or the cues to which we are responding. Moreover, we may be unconsciously responding to an action disposition that the other may be unaware of. As Brian Parkinson (1995) suggests in his review of the literature on affective communication, "Moment-by-moment reactions to another person's displays are not mediated by any conscious emotional conclusions about what these expressions signify but rather are part of one's skilled and automatized engagement in interpersonal life, and one's ecological attunement to the unfolding dynamic aspects of the situation" (p. 279).

What implications does this have for the psychotherapy process in general and for therapeutic alliance ruptures in particular? Patients and therapists are always resonating with one another at bodily-felt levels. The heart of the therapeutic process involves affective communication at both conscious and unconscious levels. This is a complex and multidimensional process. Therapists' ability to attune to their patients' unarticulated emotional experience plays a critical role in the initial development of the alliance. It also enables them to help patients articulate aspects of their affective experience that are tacit in nature. This is particularly important since affect provides information that is critical to adaptive functioning. It is also important since the symbolization of affective experience is a critical part of the process of meaning construction. Therapists' ability to attend to and symbolize their own emotional experience also allows them to elucidate the subtle and sometimes contradictory action dispositions that are evoked in them by their patients. As we shall see, this can provide a critical point of entry into unpacking and coming to understand the complex and confusing interactional processes associated with alliance ruptures. Finally, the therapists' ability to resonate with their patients' more painful emotions and to tolerate the intensely painful and frightening emotions that can be evoked in them during therapeutic alliance ruptures and treatment impasses can be transformative for patients in and of itself. As we will discuss subsequently, this type of containment (to use Bion's term), in which therapists process emotions evoked in them by patients in a nondefensive way, can be a powerful way of helping them to learn that relationships will not necessarily be destroyed by painful, aggressive, or potentially divisive feelings and that they themselves can survive these feelings.

UNDERSTANDING AND EXPERIENCING/ INSIGHT AND AWARENESS

The question of whether new *understanding* or *experiencing* is the most important mechanism of change goes back to the early days of psychoanalysis when analysts such as Ferenczi and Rank criticized Freud for intellectualist tendencies. Although in the heyday of classical analytic theory the role of new understanding was often emphasized at the expense of new experience, there has been a decisive swing in recent years to redress this imbalance (see Wallerstein, 1995). Although conceptual understanding plays an important role in helping people to change, in the absence of new experience therapy remains an intellectual exercise. New experience can take different forms.

One of the most important forms of new experience takes place through the relationship with the therapist. By working collaboratively with the patient to discover how both are contributing to the current interaction, the therapist is able to provide the patient with a new constructive interpersonal experience that challenges the patient's existing relational schemas. This basic proposition, which can be found in earliest form in Ferenczi's (1932) work, has become central to contemporary relational thinking. A second form of new experience involves the new awareness of internal experience that has previously been disowned. For example, a patient who contacts feelings of anger or sadness that have previously been disowned is provided with irrefutable evidence about an aspect of self-experience that can change his self-concept. A third form of new experience involves becoming aware of an aspect of one's actions that has previously taken place out of awareness. For example, a patient who withdraws in a self-protective fashion becomes aware of this act as it is taking place. A related form of new experience involves becoming aware of one's own defensive processes as they are taking place. For example, the intellectualizing patient becomes aware of the intellectualized avoidance of emotional experience as it is taking place. A final form of new experience involves the present awareness of some aspect of one's own construction of reality as it takes place. For example, a patient becomes aware of denigrating himself as this process is taking place.

Related to this distinction between understanding and experiencing is the distinction between *insight* and *awareness*. Awareness can be distinguished from insight in that it involves direct awareness of immediate experience or actions rather than retrospective reflection about them. While retrospective reflection about aspects of one's experience can play an important role in the change process, it is not sufficient in and of itself. It is only through the immediate awareness of experience that new possibilities emerge.

One of the problems in many discussions about the role of insight in the change process is a lack of clarity about what the term means. Most therapists agree that insight has something to do with acquiring new knowledge. The perennial question, however, is what type of knowledge acquisition is related to change? The traditional way of answering this question has involved distinguishing between intellectual and emotional insight. James Strachey (1934), for example, spoke early on about the importance of emotional immediacy in the change process. He suggested that in order to be effective, an interpretation "must be emotionally 'immediate': the patient must experience it as something actual" (p. 333). According to him, in order for the interpretation to be emotionally immediate, it must be directed at an emotional experience that is currently activated, typically in the form of a feeling that the patient has toward the therapist. Strachey's understanding of this process, however, was grounded in a drive theory that is rejected by many contemporary theorists.

The recognition that the human mind is embodied (Damasio, 1994; Gibson, 1979; Shaw & Bransford, 1977; Varela, Thompson, & Rosch, 1991; Weimer, 1977) provides an important starting point for exploring the issue in more contemporary terms. As emotion theory suggests, there is an intrinsic connection between knowledge and action. The human mind has evolved its distinctive characteristics due to their significance for adaptive action in the real world; and thinking, feeling, and acting are interdependent aspects of the same process. This contrasts with the view more commonly held in Western psychology in which the mind is seen as a type of thought machine residing in the head. Instead, thinking is understood to be an embodied process. We know things not just through our heads, but also through our actions and our bodily-felt experience.

There is an important aspect of knowledge acquisition that involves acquiring a bodily-felt sense, or what Eugene Gendlin (1991) refers to as "bodily sentience." We are constantly processing the meaning of the current situation at a bodily-felt level, and acting out of this bodily sentience in an ongoing fashion. This bodily-felt knowledge becomes integrated with higher level cognition through a complex combination of information-processing activities, and the product of this integration is the subjective experience of emotion (Greenberg & Safran, 1987; Leventhal, 1984). As previously indicated, emotion thus provides a type of integrative function, in that it integrates both higher level, more abstract cortical activity with lower level bodily sentience, or perceptual–motor behavior (see Leventhal, 1984).

This type of integration is very important. Since the process of knowing takes place at various levels, it is possible for someone to know something at one level without knowing it at another level. For example, it is possible for someone to have a bodily-felt sense of something without knowing it at a conceptual level. Albert Einstein maintained that he knew the theory of relativity at the level of gut feeling before he was able to articulate it at a mathematical and conceptual level (Holton, 1971). Some have argued that the creative process always involves taking bodily-felt knowledge and articulating it at a more conceptual level (e.g., Briggs, 1988; Polanyi, 1966).

In the clinical domain, the discrepancy between levels can result in a type of alienation from the self. For example, a patient experiences feelings of sadness or anger at a bodily-felt level, but not in conceptual awareness. In this situation, insight of a therapeutic nature, or *awareness*, would involve integrating conceptual awareness with the level of bodily-felt experience, or, to use Roy Schafer's (1983) phrase, "owning a disclaimed action." It is important to be clear that we are not suggesting that this type of integration simply involves discovering knowledge that is already present in our bodies, or of transferring information coded in one modality to another. Consistent with Gadamer's (1960) perspective, we find it more helpful to regard the new meaning that emerges out of reflecting on one's own bodily-felt experience as both discovered and constructed (see also Stern, 1997).

It is also possible to know something at a conceptual level but not at a bodily-felt level. For example, one can have an excellent understanding of the subtleties of skiing at a conceptual level and yet be a disaster on the ski slope. Of course, having a theoretical understanding of how to ski can be useful in actually learning how to ski. Ultimately, however, there is no substitute for experiential learning. One has to get the "feel" for making a well-executed parallel turn. A conceptual understanding of this process is, at best, to use Alfred Korzybski's (1933) phrase, a "map of the real territory."

Similarly, when it comes to therapy, a conceptual understanding of the way in which one constructs one's own reality through thought and action cannot by itself bring about real change. A patient can have a conceptual understanding of the way that she protects herself from abandonment, and yet not see how she is doing this in the present moment with her therapist. Ultimately, one must experience what one is doing at a bodily-felt level.

As Gendlin (1991) suggests, bodily-felt knowing is always interactional, and it always has implications for action. Unlike more conceptual thinking, which can be detached from action, bodily-felt knowing always has implications for the next step in the present. When a person has a new feeling, it provides her with irrefutable information about what the entire situational configuration really means to her as a whole organism, and this meaning has implicit implications for action. When an individual has what is traditionally referred to as "emotional insight," things are seen in a new way in a fashion that connects with current lived experience. Emotional insight or awareness thus involves reappraising an event or experience in a fashion that gets at "what this means to me now." When an individual has an emotionally immediate awareness in the present, it means that he or she is seeing things from a new perspective as a whole-integrated organism. It reflects the fact that the individual knows something differently as an embodied organism in interaction with the environment.

This type of experiential shift does not complete the change process. Rather, it establishes an experiential foundation for future moments of bodily-felt awareness in different contexts. Generalizing this awareness to other occasions is not, however, a conceptual process. It involves a discipline of maintaining awareness in the present.

PARTICIPANT-OBSERVATION
AND OBSERVING-PARTICIPATION

Harry Stack Sullivan (1965) originally borrowed the term "participant-observer" from sociology and anthropology to refer to the observational stance that the therapist should take in order to learn about the interpersonal field that is being coconstructed by the patient–therapist dyad. The need for this type of observational stance is, of course, premised on the axiom that the observer inevitably influences the observed. There is thus no such thing as a neutral, impartial observer or a phenomenon (i.e., patient) that exists and can be observed independent of the observer. Despite Sullivan's endorsement of field theory, his clinical practice nevertheless retained a positivist bent. He believed that it was possible for the therapist to take into account his or her own contribution to the interaction and in some respects to stand outside of it and function as an expert on human relations. Unlike mainstream analysts who focused on the analysis of the transference, Sullivan's focus was outside of the therapeutic relationship.

Subsequent interpersonalists, beginning with Clara Thompson (1950) and continuing with theorists such as Benjamin Wolstein (1959) and Edgar Levenson (1972), began to focus more explicitly on the here-and-now of the therapeutic relationship. In this respect, they brought interpersonal practice more in line with mainstream psychoanalysis, but with the additional innovation consisting of the recognition of the therapist's full participation in the interpersonal field. In recent years, this type of emphasis on the mutuality of the therapeutic relationship has also emerged in the work of contemporary Freudians such as Owen Renik (1995), Judith Chused (1991), and James McLaughlin (1991). Much of the contemporary Freudian emphasis on the mutuality of the therapeutic relationship appears to be crystallizing around the concept of *enactment* (e.g., Jacobs, 1986), which is seen as a two-party interactional situation deriving from unconscious sources in both patient and therapist.

While many contemporary psychoanalytic theorists converge in attributing some degree of mutuality to the therapeutic relationship, there is considerable variation in the weight given to patient versus therapist contributions and in the understanding of the extent to which the therapist can ever come to fully understand his or her own contributions. The term "observing-participant" (as opposed to participant-observer) was introduced by Erich Fromm (1964) to characterize the view that the therapist's unwitting participation in the enactment is both inevitable and desirable (see also Hirsch, 1996). Similarly, Wolstein (1975) suggested the term "coparticipant" to emphasize the same point. This view holds that countertransference is the regular state of affairs, rather than a periodic aberration, and that the therapist's understanding of the nature of his or her own participation often takes place after the fact and is at best only partial (e.g., Aron, 1996; Mitchell, 1993; Renik, 1995).

INTERSUBJECTIVITY

The movement toward a two-person psychology and the increasing attention paid to therapist experience and participation has also been marked by the proliferation of perspectives often described as "intersubjective" (see Aron, 1996), and sometimes as "subject-relations" (see Bollas, 1987; Kennedy, 1997). These perspectives represent a shift away from viewing the therapeutic relationship in terms of discrete enactments involving transference and countertransference (where the direction of influence is largely from the patient to the therapist and the implication is that what is experienced by the patient is distorted and irrational) and to viewing the relationship as an ongoing interplay of separate subjectivities. While this type of interplay of subjectivities is part of the ongoing process of treatment, it is particularly salient during the negotiation of alliance ruptures.

The notion of intersubjectivity has been articulated by various traditions and applied in a variety of ways. Based on his infant research, for example, Daniel Stern (1985) described a course of development for children whereby they achieve the capacity to recognize an other as a separate center of subjectivity with whom a subjective state can be shared. Other infant researchers, such as Beatrice Beebe and Frank Lachmann (1992), have focused on the ways in which the subjective states of mother and child are interpersonally communicated and regulated. The emphasis in their work seems to be more on mutual regulation or influence than on mutual recognition (in contrast to theorists such as Jessica Benjamin, whom we will discuss below).

In the psychotherapy literature, Robert Stolorow and colleagues (Atwood & Stolorow, 1984; Stolorow & Atwood, 1992; Stolorow, Brandchaft, & Atwood, 1994), as well as Joseph Natterson (1991), have used the idea of intersubjectivity in their extension of self psychological theory. They consider it as an overarching term to describe the psychological field between patient and therapist, that is, "the interplay between the differently organized subjective worlds" (Atwood & Stolorow, 1984, p. 41), "the reciprocal influence of the conscious and unconscious subjectivities" (Natterson, 1991, p. 1) of the two people in the relationship. As with Beebe and Lachman, the emphasis here is on mutual regulation.

Jessica Benjamin's (1988, 1990) notion of intersubjectivity integrates a number of perspectives and provides a comprehensive view of mutual recognition and regulation in the psychotherapeutic situation. Influenced by feminist psychoanalytic criticism, Benjamin challenges the traditional psychoanalytic view of the mother as an object to the infant's drives and needs. She argues that the child must recognize the mother as a separate subject with her own experiential world, intentions, and desires, and that the capacity for such recognition is a developmental achievement. Adapting Freud's oft-quoted statement about the aim of psychoanalysis, she suggests, "Where objects were, subjects must be" (1990, p. 34).

One can clearly see in her ideas about the analytic situation the influence of critical theorists like Jürgen Habermas (1971), who used the term "intersubjectivity" in contrasting subject–subject relations to subject–object relations. One can also see the influence of Dorothy Dinnerstein (1976), who wrote: "Every 'I' first emerges in relation to an 'It' which is not at all clearly an 'I.' The separate 'I'ness of the other person is a discovery, an insight achieved over time" (p. 106). These perspectives, in turn, echo Martin Buber's (1923) "interhuman" philosophy of dialogue, as well as ideas from Hegel (1807). Buber contrasted what he referred to as the "I–Thou" relationship with the "I–It" relationship. The I–Thou relationship involves the recognition of the other as a subject. It is characterized by mutuality, directness, presentness, and the absence of contrivance. In contrast, the I–It relationship involves relating to the other as an object. It is characterized by a lack of mutuality and presentness; the other is related to in terms of preexisting categories, rather than in his or her own terms. Buber suggested that mutual recognition of separate subjectivities, his I–Thou relation, coexists in dialectic with the subject–object, I–It relation. Both are necessary in human relationships.

According to Hegel (1807), self-consciousness or the experience of oneself as a self can only emerge through the recognition of the other. Without this recognition, I can experience events, but can have no experience of myself as an experiencing agent. We are thus fundamentally dependent upon others for the experience of selfhood. Thus the other is a danger to me because he threatens my self-sufficiency. It is for this reason that what Hegel refers to as the "master–slave conflict" begins. The master–slave dialectic plays out as follows. Because I do not wish to be dependent upon the other's recognition for my sense of self, I try to control him or her. The other is simultaneously trying to control me in order to preserve his or her own freedom as a self-sufficient consciousness. I can assume one of two positions in this struggle. Either I can assume the position of the master, thereby controlling the other, or I can assume the position of the slave, thereby allowing the other to control me. The problem is that neither of these positions is satisfactory. If I assume the position of the slave, I am only important insofar as I am important to the other. I thus have no freedom of existence or ability to define myself. If, however, I assume the position of the master, I deprive the other of the independent existence necessary to confirm my existence as a subject. Thus, there is a supreme irony here in that to the extent that we succeed in obtaining our goal of possessing or controlling others (or at least deceiving ourselves into believing that we do), we increase our sense of aloneness.

Unlike Stern, Benjamin considers the developmental achievement of intersubjectivity (i.e., the recognition of the subjectivity of the other) as one that is inconsistently maintained. Influenced by D. W. Winnicott (1965), as well as by Buber (1923) and Hegel (1807), she argues that the therapeutic situation must invariably involve a dialectical tension between relating to the other as an object and relating to the other as a subject. This process continually involves both the recognition and negation of the other as a separate center of subjectivity. Influenced by Winnicott's (1969) thinking, Benjamin argues that the ability to use the other as an object of one's aggression ultimately plays a role in helping one to experience the other as an independent subject (see Chapter 3).

In a related vein, Lewis Aron (1996) has described intimacy in a dyadic encounter as dependent upon the mutual recognition of each other's separate subjectivity, but not coterminous with it (see Ehrenberg, 1992; Singer, 1977; Wilner, 1975; Wolstein, 1994). For Aron, "Intimacy involves the survival and sustenance of a relation through the ongoing creation and destruction of intersubjectivity. . . . It requires mutual openness, mutual directness, interaffectivity, and personal exposure and risk" (1996, p. 152). As we will discuss in Chapter 3, during alliance ruptures, the therapist's ability to survive patients' aggression and work through their disappointments can play a critical role in helping them to experience others as subjects. This helps them both to become more accepting of others' limitations and more self-accepting.

MINDFULNESS: THE THERAPIST'S
OBSERVATIONAL STANCE AND INNER WORK

Given the pivotal role that the therapist's observational stance plays in the therapeutic enterprise, it is striking how little has been written about it. Freud's (1912) assertion that the therapist should listen to his or her patient with "evenly hovering attention" has been accepted as a cornerstone by subsequent psychoanalytic theorists, and for this reason it is worth quoting him at length.

> It . . . consists in making no effort to concentrate the attention on anything in particular, and maintaining in regard to all that one hears the same measure of calm, quiet attentiveness—of "evenly-hovering attention." . . . As soon as attention is deliberately concentrated in a certain degree, one begins to select from the material before one; one point will be fixed in the mind with particular clearness and some other consequently disregarded, and in this selection one's expectations or one's inclinations will be followed. This is just what must not be done. . . . If one's expectations are followed in this selection there is the danger of never finding anything but what is already known, and if one follows one's inclinations anything which is to be perceived will most certainly be falsified. (pp. 111–112)

This prescription is very much consistent with the state of mind referred to earlier as "beginner's mind." The emphasis is on "courting surprise" (Stern, 1997) by not allowing one's expectations to direct one's attention toward a selected aspect of the material. Despite the value of Freud's prescription, it has certain limitations from the standpoint of contemporary clinical practice. The first is that it fails to provide an adequate specification of the internal processes through which a state of evenly hovering attention can be attained. The second is that, in keeping with Freud's positioning within a one-person psychology, the focus of observation is the patient, rather than the patient–therapist dyad. In other words, it is not consistent with the stance of observant-participation or, for that matter, participant-observation.

Theodore Reik (1948), perhaps more than any other theorist, attempted to elaborate Freud's thinking on evenly hovering attention into a more comprehensive position on the therapist's listening stance. And yet, for reasons that are not entirely clear, he has been by-and-large ignored in the contemporary psychoanalytic literature. Following Freud, he argued for the importance of not allowing the attention to become attached to any one aspect of the observational field, since this limits the therapist's ability to perceive other potentially important data that are not the focus of attention. Furthermore, he highlighted the importance of suspending critical judgment in order to allow fleeting impressions to emerge into awareness. Finally, he emphasized that it was critical for therapists to turn their attention inward in order to attend to relevant data emerging from their own experience. He argued that many of the more subtle nuances of interpersonal communication are both expressed and perceived at unconscious levels, and that only by looking inward and listening with the "third ear" could the therapist come to really understand his or her patients.

Although Paula Heimann (1950) is conventionally considered to be one of the more important pioneers to focus on the role of unconscious communication between patient and therapist, Reik actually explored this phenomenon in considerably more detail and provided numerous illuminating clinical illustrations of the way in which the therapist can deepen his or her understanding of the patient by attending to fleeting impressions, feelings, images, and fantasies that are on the edge of his or her own awareness.

As previously mentioned, Wilfred Bion's (1967) article "Notes on Memory and Desire" was an important attempt to further articulate the nature of the therapist's observational stance (see also Bion, 1970). The essence of Bion's position was that every session with the patient must be approached as if it were the first one, since to assimilate one's understanding of the patient into what is already "known" about him or her, or into one's theories, will prevent the therapist from being open to new possibilities as they emerge. Furthermore, he argued that the therapist must let go of his or her desire to obtain any objective, since this will cloud his or her vision and prevent him or her from relating fully to the immediacy of the moment. While Bion's recommendations are important, they are written in an aphoristic fashion, without any articulation of how this ideal stance can be attained.

More recently, Donnel Stern (1997) has applied Gadamer's hermeneutic perspective to psychoanalysis in a creative fashion to emphasize the point that real understanding can only take place when the therapist works to illuminate and challenge his or her own preconceptions through "genuine conversation" with the patient. His focus, however, is on describing the relevant observational stance in general terms, rather than on articulating the associated internal processes.

Thomas Ogden (1994) has written in a particularly intriguing fashion about the way in which the therapist can attend to his or her own inner associations to the patient's material in order to deepen his or her understanding of the patient. He invokes the concept of "the analytic third" to account for the informational value of the therapist's fleeting associations, images, and fantasies. According to him, the analytic third is a third subject in the room that is constituted by the joint contributions of patient and therapist. The therapist's inner experience will inevitably be influenced by this analytic third and thus will inevitably say something about both therapist and patient.

Another important contemporary exploration of the role that the therapist's inner work can play in the therapeutic process can be found in the writing of Theodore Jacobs (1991). He provides compelling accounts of the way in which the therapist can gain an empathic understanding of the patient's inner struggles by engaging in a type of inner work through which personal memories, emotions, and shifting self-states that are evoked by and resonate with the patient's inner struggles are reflected on. In Jacobs's approach, this type of reflection takes place internally and is not shared with the patient.

The above recommendations on the therapist's observational stance can be further fleshed out and amplified through the literature on mindfulness that has emerged from Buddhist psychology. The Buddhist tradition of mindfulness is a highly sophisticated method of self-exploration, which can be adapted in order to help therapists cultivate the stance of participant-observation (Epstein, 1995; Rubin, 1996). In contrast to the relatively sparse psychoanalytic literature detailing the process involved in cultivating the therapist's observational stance, the literature on mindfulness is vast, and there are numerous detailed and systematic technical treatises on how to develop and implement the skill of mindfulness, some dating back as far as the first century B.C.E.

The tradition of mindfulness contains another element that is consistent with the needs of the therapist practicing with the sensibility of a participant-observer. The emphasis in mindfulness is not just on the observation of one's internal experience in specific settings but also on mindfulness in action. Although the most well-known mindfulness exercises involve meditating while sitting, the general emphasis is on integrating mindfulness into everyday life, and a variety of different strategies are taught for doing this (such as practicing while walking or engaging in everyday activities, like eating or working).

Mindfulness involves directing one's attention in order to become aware of one's thoughts, feelings, fantasies, or actions as they take place in the present moment. The goal of mindfulness is to become aware of and then to deautomate our habitual ways of structuring our experience through automatic psychological activities and actions. It has important parallels with both Freud's evenly hovering attention and with Richard Sterba's observing ego.

Mindfulness involves three components: (1) the direction of attention, (2) remembering, and (3) nonjudgmental awareness. The initial direction of attention involves intentionally paying attention to and observing one's inner experience or actions. This involves cultivating an attitude of intense curiosity about one's experience. In mindfulness meditation, the individual can initially cultivate the ability to attend by focusing the attention on an object (e.g., the breath), and then noting whenever his or her attention has wandered and returning it to the intended focus of attention. By noting whatever one's attention has wandered toward (e.g., a particular thought or feeling), before redirecting one's attention, the individual develops the ability to observe and investigate his or her experience from a detached perspective rather than being fully immersed in or identified with it.

The component of remembering plays a crucial role in allowing the individual to become aware of when he or she has lost the stance of the detached observer by becoming absorbed in a particular thought, feeling, or fantasy without awareness. It is anticipated that people's attention will constantly flit around from focus to focus, and that they will become lost in the objects of their attention (e.g., fantasies, memories, pleasant and painful feelings) on an ongoing basis. Once again, the task is to periodically become aware of the object, thereby allowing it to dissolve, and to then return one's attention to a poised or evenly hovering position.

The component of nonjudgmental awareness plays a critical role in helping people to observe whatever emerges without pushing it out of awareness and without losing the stance of mindfulness, by getting caught up in an infinite spiral of self-judgment. Although the suspension of critical judgment is considered essential, it is recognized that it is inevitable that the individual will at times feel critical of his or her own experience or of others. The task is thus not to completely eliminate critical judgment, but to become aware of it as it emerges. This process of awareness then allows the judgment to dissolve, by making it fully conscious, thereby depriving it of its power and freeing up attention once again. *At the most fundamental level, what emerges as particularly critical to the stance of mindfulness is this attitude of acceptance.* Objects of attention can never be forcefully pushed out of awareness without creating an internal struggle that will only make them more powerful. Only the act of accepting awareness deprives the contents of the mind of their force.

An important by-product of mindfulness practice is the discovery of *internal space*. This consists of a loosening of attachment to one's cognitive–affective processes—an ability to see them as constructions of the mind. This in turn reduces the experience of constriction resulting from overidentification with these processes and allows one to reflect on them and use them therapeutically. This experience is similar to what theorists, such as Thomas Ogden (1986) and Glen Gabbard (1996), refer to as *analytic space*, that is, the state of "double consciousness" that allows therapists to be "sucked into the patient's world while still maintaining their observing capacity" (Gabbard & Wilkinson, 1994, p. 87).

CIRCLES, CYCLES, AND MATRICES

The question of why people persist in self-defeating patterns has always been a perplexing one for psychotherapy theorists. A central theme in the thinking of interpersonal and relational theorists is that people inevitably perceive and shape new relationships according to prestructured notions about how people connect. These prestructured notions are derived from previous interpersonal experience. The idea that people have a primary motivation for human relatedness dates back to the work of Sandor Ferenczi and Michael Balint and was developed more fully in the work of theorists such as W. R. D. Fairbairn and Harry Stack Sullivan.

Given the importance for survival purposes of maintaining relatedness to others, particularly in infants, it is adaptive to represent past experience in a way that maximizes this possibility. Consistent with this line of reasoning, John Bowlby (1969, 1973, 1980) theorized that human beings develop internal working models representing interpersonal interactions relevant to attachment behavior. This type of working model can be thought of as an *interpersonal* or *relational schema* (Safran, 1984, 1990a, 1998; Baldwin, 1992) that is abstracted on the basis of interactions with attachment figures and that permits the individual to predict interactions in a way that increases the probability of maintaining relatedness with these figures. It is a representation of self–other relationships, rather than a representation of self or a representation of other. It is thus intrinsically interactional in nature (a view that was anticipated by Fairbairn, 1952). In Daniel Stern's (1985) terms, a relational schema consists of representations of interactions that have been generalized (RIGs).

As Bowlby (1969) maintains, animals of every species are genetically biased to respond with anxiety to stimulus situations that serve as naturally occurring cues to events potentially dangerous to that species. Because maintaining proximity to other human beings plays such an important role in the survival of the human species (particularly in the helpless infant who depends upon the caretaker for moment-by-moment survival), it is not surprising that the perception of a potential disruption in an interpersonal relationship would automatically elicit an anxiety response in human beings. It is thus reasonable to hypothesize that human beings are by nature perceptually attuned to detect any cues regarding the potential disintegration of interpersonal relationships and are programmed to respond with anxiety. Anxiety serves as a cue function in that behaviors and experiences that become associated with the disruption or disintegration of relationships with significant others also become identified as dangerous and subsequently trigger anxiety.

Although Fairbairn's object relational perspective shares much with Bowlby's model of attachment, Fairbairn adds to Bowlby's ethological perspective on attachment as automatic and reflexive by highlighting the role of desire and affect. He vividly portrays the hunger for attachment, the longing for connection, and the loyalty to old object ties that propel human relations (see Mitchell, 1988, for an elaboration).

According to Sullivan (1953, 1956), we come to experience certain personal characteristics belonging to the self through the reflected appraisals of others. Those characteristics that are valued by significant others become personified as the self (the "good me" in Sullivan's terms), and positively valued, whereas those experiences and characteristics that are associated with a moderate degree of disruption in significant interpersonal relationships (and thus with a moderate degree of anxiety) still become personified as part of the self, but come to be viewed negatively. Sullivan referred to these feelings, experiences, and characteristics as the "bad me." At the extreme end of the continuum are feelings, characteristics, and experiences that have in the past been associated with severe disruption in significant interpersonal relationships. Because of the intense anxiety associated with these experiences, the processing of information around them, both external (reactions of others) and internal (thoughts and feelings), is obstructed, and such information is not well coded in memory. For this reason, experiences and characteristics associated with extreme anxiety do not become well integrated in memory with other information, and do not become represented as part of the self. Sullivan referred to experiences and characteristics of this kind as the "not me." It is important to keep in mind that these different aspects of the self are not static, discontinuous structures, but rather continuous shifting aspects of experience that are influenced by the current relational context.

Relational schemas shape the way that people relate to both their inner and outer worlds on an ongoing basis. They represent the bases for the intrapsychic and interpersonal patterns that we repeatedly en-act, patterns that others have referred to as *vicious circles* (Horney, 1950; Strachey, 1934; Wachtel, 1997) and that we have previously described as *cognitive-interpersonal cycles* (e.g., Safran, 1984b; Safran, 1990a, 1990b; Safran & Segal, 1990). Stephen Mitchell (1988) uses the term *relational matrix* to refer to the individual's self-perpetuating cycle of internal representations, actions, and characteristic actions of others. These relational schemas structure our relationships with other people in a number of ways:

1. People act in accordance with a rigid self-definition in order to maintain relatedness with others. For example, the individual who has learned that relatedness is contingent on being helpful and responsive to others' needs may consistently adopt the helping role in his relationships with others. He will select friends and intimates who are comfortable playing the reciprocal role, and socialize others into expecting him to play that role. As a result he is unlikely to establish relationships with people who are comfortable responding to his own emotional needs, and this will confirm his belief that he needs to be a "helper" in order to maintain relatedness.

2. People act in a characteristic fashion in response to the failings of others that they anticipate and elicit. For example, the individual who anticipates others to be hostile will have a readiness to interpret actions as hostile and act with preemptive and self-protective hostility, thereby eliciting the hostility that is expected. This evokes anger in other people, thereby confirming his expectation of abandonment.

3. People who believe that relatedness is contingent on a mode of being consistent with a rigid self-definition dissociate aspects of their experience consistent with that self-definition. Dissociated aspects of self-experience are nevertheless expressed through one's nonverbal behavior and actions. The resulting incongruent communication results in characteristic responses from others that confirm one's expectations of self–other interactions (the relational configuration the individual expects). For example, the individual who dissociates angry feelings will nevertheless communicate anger through her actions and through subtleties of her nonverbal behavior. Other people will respond to the dissociated anger that is being communicated with their own anger, often without being aware of what they are responding to. There is thus a mystification that takes place in the relationship, which leaves both partners in the interaction confused about what is going on (Laing, 1969; Levenson, 1992). The individual who dissociates his anger experiences himself as victimized and unjustly attacked by the individual who responds to his dissociated anger. This intensifies his own

feelings of hurt and anger, which continue to be dissociated and communicated in incongruent and disclaimed form. The individual who responds to the incongruent communication may leave the interaction as confused as the first person.

4. When people have incipient feelings or thoughts that are experienced as threatening to relatedness, they attempt to manage them through defensive operations. These defensive operations in turn elicit certain predictable reactions from others that confirm their working models of self–other interactions. For example, the individual who anticipates that an other will abandon him when he is vulnerable, defends against his sadness and presents a calm and rational front. This distances people and reduces the possibility that they will respond in a nurturing fashion. This in turn confirms his belief that vulnerable feelings are unacceptable.

BEYOND COUNTERTRANSFERENCE

Over time, an important shift has taken place in the psychoanalytic perspective on countertransference. Freud (1910) originally conceptualized countertransference feelings as the therapist's unconscious reactions to the patients, reflecting personal conflicts in the therapist that need to be resolved. Countertransference feelings were thus viewed as obstacles to therapy that need to be overcome. This perspective on countertransference, referred to as the "classical perspective" by Otto Kernberg (1965), has increasingly given way to what he refers to as the "totalist perspective." The totalist perspective holds that countertransference feelings can provide the therapist with important information about the patient. As previously mentioned, Paula Heimann (1950) is credited as being one of the first to recognize the potential value of the therapist's countertransference feelings as an important source of information about the patient. She believed that the therapist's unconscious understanding of the patient is superior to his or her conscious understanding, and further believed that by attending to feelings evoked within by the patient, he or she could gain access to this unconscious understanding. Although she did not believe in actually sharing feelings evoked in therapy with the patient, others, such as Margaret Little (1951) and Winnicott (1947), did advocate the judicious disclosure of countertransference feelings.

Heinrich Racker (1953, 1968) wrote extensively about the therapeutic use of countertransference feelings and argued that every transference situation provokes a corresponding countertransference response. According to him, countertransference feelings can reflect the therapist's identification with the patient's internalized objects or with unconscious aspects of the patient's self, and as such can provide important information about the patient. He believed that failure to become aware of one's countertransference feelings leads to a repetition of the vicious circle that is characteristic for the patient, whereas awareness of one's countertransference feelings can lead to a deeper understanding of the patient. Racker was less detailed in his consideration of countertransference disclosure, though he could imagine some situations in which it would be of value. Other notable proponents of a totalist perspective on countertransference historically were Ralph Greenson (1974), Joseph Sandler (1976), and Merton Gill (1982).

In recent years, it has become increasingly common to understand countertransference in terms of the concept of projective identification. Although Melanie Klein (1975) originally used the concept to refer exclusively to the patient's intrapsychic processes, subsequent Kleinians, particularly Bion (1962), elaborated the concept in a more interpersonal direction. Ogden (1979), among others, has played an important role in popularizing the concept of projective identification in North American circles. Common to most conceptualizations of projective identification is the view that the patient projects unwanted aspects of the self onto the therapist and in one way or another nudges or coerces the therapist into experiencing the disowned feelings and into acting in accordance with the projection. If the therapist is able to contain the projection and metabolize the experience (to use Money-Kyrle's [1956] metaphor), the patient is able to recover the disowned aspects of the self in detoxified form. Moreover, the thinking is that since the therapist's feelings can be projected into him by the patient, they can provide an invaluable source of information about inchoate feelings that the patient dissociates and that could not otherwise be accessed.

The following example, condensed from Ogden (1982), provides an illustration of the therapeutic use of the concept of projective identification:

> Mr. C., a 29-year-old married man, worked as a stockbroker. At the beginning of the second month of treatment, a senior member of the brokerage house where the patient was working, who had been a mentor to Mr. C., left the firm for another job. At around the same time, the therapist noticed that Mr. C. began to fill each session with an ongoing monologue that had the effect of crowding the therapist out. In the next few weeks, Mr. C. began to talk about his fantasies that the therapist was not particularly competent or successful. He also began to denigrate the therapist in other ways, such as by telling him that he felt "very macho" and athletic com-

pared to the therapist, and that he imagined he could beat him at any sport. Mr. C. admitted that he felt guilty and afraid of hurting the therapist, but the pattern nevertheless continued.

The therapist became increasingly aware of his own feelings of impotence, and reflected to himself that his own feelings of inadequacy vis-à-vis his own father were probably being rekindled through the interaction with his patient. However, as the therapist "thought more about the changes that had taken place in the patient over the previous two months, and the powerful feelings of inadequacy and emasculation, he began to consider the possibility that his own feelings had been to a large extent evoked by the patient as a component of a projective identification that involved the patient's feelings of inadequacy in relation to a paternal transference figure" (p. 49). This understanding of the situation was facilitated by the therapist's knowledge that the patient's father had indeed been overbearing.

According to Ogden, conceptualizing what was taking place in terms of projective identification provided the therapist with the psychological room he needed to reflect more carefully on the nature of what was being enacted in the relationship. Prior to understanding the nature of the projection, the therapist's intense feelings of inadequacy and shame prevented him from working productively. However, argues Ogden, "the perspective of projective identification allowed the therapist to make use of his feeling-state to inform his understanding of the transference, and not simply to further his understanding of himself or to prevent his own conflicts from interfering with the therapy" (p. 49). The therapist began to consider the possibility that his own feelings of inadequacy were a projection of the patient's conflictual feelings of dependency and inadequacy in relation to father figures. These, he speculated, were triggered by the departure of the patient's mentor and played out in the transference relationship.

There are a variety of criticisms of the concept of projective identification from a more purist interpersonal perspective. Aron (1996) views the extension of the concept projective identification in a more interpersonal direction as a rhetorical strategy that permits the recognition of interactive elements within orthodox (and traditionally one-person psychology) psychoanalytic theory. Another criticism concerns the ambiguity and lack of conceptual clarity regarding both the intrapsychic and the interpersonal processes believed to underlie the mechanism. A third criticism is that the concept can easily be used to disclaim the therapist's responsibility for her role in the interaction. The idea that feelings can be "put into" the therapist by the patient can lead to blaming the patient for distressing feelings, rather than attempting to understand one's own contribution. Proponents of the concept are increasingly sensitive to this danger and emphasize that the projection can never simply be put into the therapist, but must interact with and activate something already existing in the therapist before it takes final form (e.g., Joseph, 1989; Gabbard, 1995).

The concept does not have to be used in a defensive fashion and can have clinical utility. It can provide a conceptual framework that can help the therapist manage the anxiety associated with distressing feelings and reorient him or her toward those feelings with an attitude of therapeutic curiosity. Nevertheless, there is something intrinsic to the concept that lends itself to being used defensively or at least to squeezing the complexities of lived experience into a prestructured formulation. The use of the concept can result in the type of reification described earlier.

While in some cases the therapist's feelings can provide an important clue to inchoate aspects of the patient's experience, the practice of moving directly from one's own experience to inferring disowned aspects of the patient's experience forecloses the exploration of the subtleties of the relational matrix that mediate the process. (But see Stephen Seligman, 1999, for a recent attempt to integrate the use of the concept of projective identification with a more nuanced exploration of the relevant interactive matrix.) For example, in the illustration taken from Ogden (1982), what was going on for Mr. C. when he began crowding his therapist out with a verbal barrage? Was he feeling vulnerable and afraid of being impinged upon by his therapist? Was he feeling helpless and afraid of showing his need for fear that the therapist would abandon him or control him? Was he feeling angry and afraid of showing it? How did Mr. C. perceive his therapist and react to his therapist's reaction? To what extent was he consciously aware of his therapist's feelings of inadequacy? How did he feel about any perception of such feelings that he registered either consciously or unconsciously? Was the therapist feeling resentful at all? If so, how conscious was the patient of these feelings, and how did he feel about them?

Alternatives to conceptualizing the transference–countertransference matrix in terms of projective identification are notions such as Edgar Levenson's (1972) *transformation* or Joseph Sandler's (1976) idea of *role responsiveness*. These perspectives suggest that patients approach their relationships with others with characteristic ways of organizing experience that impact upon their actions and elicit predictable reactions from others (see Strupp & Binder, 1984). As Mitchell (1988) puts it, the therapist, like any other human being, inevitably becomes embedded in the patient's relational matrix. The therapist's task is not one of avoiding or managing countertransference feelings, but one of using her experience of engagement in the patient's relational matrix to come to understand who the patient is in the world. Therapists thus cannot but be embedded in this matrix, nor should they try to avoid it (Kiesler, 1996; Kiesler, & Watkins, 1989). Premature attempts to avoid embeddedness will prevent them from coming to understand the way that they are embedded and will rob them of the most important information available to them. Moreover, therapists may need to resemble their patients' attachment figures in some respects. As Jay Greenberg (1986) suggests, therapists may have to be sufficiently like old objects for their patients in order for core relational themes to emerge in the therapeutic relationship and be worked through in a new way.

By engaging in a collaborative exploration with the patient, the therapist has the opportunity of working her way out of her embedded position and providing the patient with a new, constructive relational experience. The task is not, as a classical psychoanalytic perspective would have it, to interpret the patient's distortion of the therapist, but rather to come to understand, to use Edgar Levenson's (1985) phrase, "What's going on around here?" The therapist's task is to work collaboratively with the patient to explore the subtleties of the interaction between the patient and the therapist and the way in which the patient's psychological structures and processes contribute to these relational patterns. This helps to demystify what is transpiring in the interpersonal field. The patient's inner world and characteristic relational patterns are two sides of the same coin, and the exploration of one side of the coin facilitates the exploration of the other.

The therapist can function as a participant-observer, who responds to the patient's interpersonal pull like others, yet is able to develop some awareness of the nature of his or her own participation. His task is to attempt to elucidate and make explicit important aspects of the affective communication taking place in the therapeutic relationship, that is, to monitor his or her own feelings, response tendencies, and actions and to use them to help identify eliciting patient actions and communications. This helps the therapist to assess the nature of the relational configuration and to pinpoint specific acts and communications that play a role in it. These pinpointed acts and communications can be thought of as *interpersonal markers* indicating useful points for exploring the patient's inner experience (Safran, 1984a, 1990a; Safran & Segal, 1990). These interpersonal markers indicate unique and ideal junctures for intrapsychic exploration since it is likely that the occurrence of those interactional patterns that are most characteristically problematic for the patient will be accompanied by those intrapsychic processes that play a pivotal role in the patient's relational matrix. They are thus the other side of the coin to the patient's internal world and an important point of intersection between the internal and external.

Identifying these interpersonal markers also helps the therapist to reflect more deeply on the subtle nuances of his or her own experience. For example, awareness of a subtle communication of anger on the patient's part may help the therapist become aware of her own anger. Identification of a subtle way in which a patient communicates dependency can help the therapist become more aware of some of the reasons underlying his feelings of inadequacy.

In the illustration taken from Ogden (1982), Mr. C.'s initial shift into a monologue that crowded the therapist out would be an important interpersonal marker to explore. In addition, both his denigration of the therapist and his confessions of guilt would be important interpersonal markers to explore. Moreover, the question arises as to whether there were other more subtle interpersonal markers that contributed to the therapist's overall sense of inadequacy and shame. Perhaps a particular voice tone or the way he looked at the therapist? Perhaps some aspect of his body posture? It is possible that a more detailed identification of relevant interpersonal markers would provide the therapist with a window into understanding Mr. C.'s inner word in a more textured fashion, and constitute a useful step in the process of clarifying and understanding the therapist's own complex and contradictory feelings, in a more nuanced fashion.

MULTIPLE SELVES

There is a growing trend in contemporary psychological and philosophical thinking to regard the experience of a bounded unitary self as an illusion, as socially and historically constructed. This perspective holds that although people experience themselves as unitary and unchanging, they in reality consist of multiple selves or multiple self-states, which possess varying degrees of compatibility with one another (e.g., Bromberg, 1996; Mitchell, 1992, 1993; Pizer, 1996). Different self-states become dominant at different times, depending upon the focus of the individual's attention. Moreover, different self-states emerge in different relational contexts. As Stern (1997) has described, we not only move in and out of self-states based on the interpersonal world we face, but we also are moved in and out of self-states by this world.

This perspective of multiple selves provides a way of viewing the intersection between interpersonal and intrapsychic realms in therapy in terms of the mutual influence of shifting self-states in patient and therapist. From this perspective, each individual experiences a perpetual cycling between different self-states, which in turn evoke complementary self-states in the other (Bach, 1994; Bromberg, 1995; Muran, 1997, in press). Thus, for example, a patient experiences a state of sadness, which triggers a fear of being vulnerable and taken advantage of, which in turn leads to an avoidant state of stoicism. The state of sadness evokes a state of caring and nurturance in the therapist, who responds empathically. This begins to heighten the patient's awareness of her own longing for nurturance, which intensifies her fear of abandonment and fuels the transition to a state of stoicism. This evokes a state of indifference in the therapist, which evokes a self-state of anger and resentment in the patient. During therapeutic impasses, it can be particularly useful to attend to reciprocal sequences of self-state transitions in the patient–therapist system.

The transitions or boundaries between self-states are often marked by changes in patients' vocal quality, facial expression, focus and content of verbal reports, emotional involvement, and so forth. As Philip Bromberg (1996) has noted, they are also marked by shifts in therapists' subjective experience of the relationship:

> No matter how important the manifest verbal content appears to be at a given moment, the analyst should try to remain simultaneously attuned to his subjective experience of the relationship and its shifting quality. . . . He should try to be experientially accessible to (1) the impact of those moments in which he becomes aware that a shift in self-state (either his own or his patient's) has taken place, and (2) the details of his own self-reflection on whether to process this awareness with his patient or to process it alone—and if with his patient, when and how to do it. (p. 520)

The "multiple selves" perspective holds that there is no central executive control in the form of the ego. Consciousness is a function of a coalition of different self-states. It is thus an emergent product of a self-organizing system. The bifurcation of the psychic system into conscious and unconscious is overly simplified and overly static. That which is conscious is that which is attended to. Attention to different self-states in different moments is a function of different stimulus cues, both internal and external.

Bromberg (1996) describes "a view of the self as decentered and the mind as a configuration of shifting, nonlinear, discontinuous states of consciousness in an ongoing dialectic with the healthy illusion of unitary selfhood" (p. 512). Sheldon Bach (1985, 1994), likewise, has paid close attention to multiplicity or what he calls "alternate states of consciousness," including their rhythmicities and transitions. They both describe an ideal psyche in which the transitions between states are relatively seamless and barely beyond awareness. Bach (1994) considers the continual cycling of states of consciousness as necessary for the maintenance of normal mental functioning in much the same way "as perpetual eye movements serve to keep the retina refreshed" and "immobilization leads to disturbances of vision" (p. 115).

As previously indicated, the particular configuration of one's self-experience is always selective. At any point in time certain aspects of self experience are predominant and others not. It is inevitable that certain aspects of self-experience will be out of focal awareness when others are dominant. In addition, certain aspects of the self will be kept out of awareness through dissociative processes. This dissociative exclusion of aspects of self from focal awareness is a form of selective inattention, similar in nature to Sullivan's understanding of the way in which security operations function. There is no ego that represses unacceptable impulses, but rather a systemic direction of attention away from those aspects of self-experience that are assessed to be potentially dangerous. Those aspects of self-experience that are dissociated are typically those that have been associated with traumatic experience of one kind or another. The relevant trauma can range from physical or sexual abuse at one end of the spectrum to experiences that have involved disruption of relatedness to parents and other attachment figures at the other end. Experiencing and accepting the multiplicity of self is part of the change process. Therapy does not entail integrating different parts of the self, but rather bringing them into dialogue with each other through awareness. As Bromberg (1993) puts it, "Health is the ability to stand in the spaces between realities without losing any of them—the capacity to feel like one self while being many" (p. 166).

An even more radical perspective on this issue can be found in the Buddhist psychology of self. Similar to postmodern thinking, Buddhist theory holds that the experience of a unitary, static self is an illusion. Rather than postulating the existence of multiple selves, however, it holds that the experience of self is constructed on a moment-by-moment basis. The self is, therefore, a process rather than a substantial entity. In this perspective, change takes place, not through facilitating dialogue between different aspects of the self, but through letting go of one's defensive need to view oneself as static and unchanging. Psychological health is synonymous with the capacity to *let go* and simply *be*, rather than striving to be anything in particular.

THE PARADOX OF ACCEPTANCE

Acceptance lies at the heart of the change process. The patient comes to therapy out of a desire to be different; yet this very desire is the source of the patient's pain. The central paradox of the human change process is that it is only by letting go of our attempts to be something we are not that change can take place. Change thus involves an act of surrender, rather than self-manipulation. A classic Zen story illustrates this point. One day a well-known Zen teacher came upon a student sitting intently in meditation. "Why are you meditating?" asked the teacher, and the student replied, "To become enlightened." At this point the teacher picked up a tile and began to polish it with a cloth. Intrigued by his behavior, the student asked, "Why are you polishing the tile?" "In order to turn it into a mirror," replied the teacher. Puzzled, the student then asked him, "How can you turn a tile into a mirror by polishing it?" And the teacher responded, "How can you turn yourself into an enlightened being by meditating?" It was at this point that the student became enlightened.

A critical therapeutic task thus consists of helping patients let go of their attempts at self-manipulation and to accept themselves. A central problem, however, consists of the fact that it is inevitable that therapists will at times become accomplices in their patients' own games of trying to improve themselves. There is something intrinsic to the structure of the therapeutic process that conflicts with the therapist's need to accept the patient. Lawrence Friedman (1988) argues that the conflicting needs for the therapist to accept the patient on his or her own terms, while at the same time not settling for these terms, is a central paradox of therapy. According to him, if the therapist "does not accept the patient on his own terms, it is as though he is asking him to be someone else; the patient will have no cause for hope, and he will not recognize the analyst's vision. If the analyst settles for the patient's terms, he is . . . betraying the patient's wish for greater fulfillment" (1988, p. 34). By virtue of the fact that therapists want to help their patients change and have a preference for some way of being for them rather than others, there is a level at which patients are not fully accepted. Regardless of how hard therapists try to be accepting, by preferring one way of being over another (e.g., being emotionally honest rather than defensive), they inevitably convey to their patients a certain lack of acceptance.

In many cases, this does not create an insurmountable problem. Despite this inherent lack of acceptance, patients can feel respected enough by their therapists and trust them sufficiently to begin acknowledging the unacceptable parts of themselves and thus to begin changing. When, however, the particular chemistry of the patient and the therapist leads to the patient feeling not sufficiently accepted, an impasse ensues. Although the therapist can at one level be very accepting of the patient, nevertheless, the implicit demand for change that the patient feels can impede change.

At such times, it is only by recognizing and accepting the fact that they are not being fully accepting of their patients that therapists can begin to become more accepting. Just as patients cannot change by forcing themselves to be one way rather than another, therapists cannot will themselves into a more accepting stance. It is here that the discipline of mindfulness becomes critical. It is vital in these situations that therapists strive to become more fully aware of the subtle and not-so-subtle aspects of nonacceptance in their attitudes and actions. In such situations, it can be helpful for therapists to acknowledge the aspect of nonacceptance in their attitudes to their patients as a first step. By commenting on the bind explicitly, an element of acceptance is introduced, and the situation begins to evolve. By acknowledging what has been taking place implicitly, the therapist becomes accepting of the part of himself that has been judgmental, and an experience of release or surrender begins to emerge. As therapists begin to acknowledge and accept their lack of acceptance and the impact it has on their patients, they are better able to appreciate their dilemmas and are able to develop a more compassionate stance toward them.

In order to facilitate this process, it is critical for therapists to cultivate their own self-acceptance. To the extent that one has difficulty accepting oneself, one will have difficulty accepting others. For example, a therapist who has difficulty accepting feelings of vulnerability in himself will have difficulties accepting feelings of vulnerability in his patient. The therapist who has difficulty accepting feelings of anger in herself will have difficulty accepting feelings of anger in her patient. The therapist who has difficulty accepting feelings of despair in himself will have difficulty accepting feelings of despair in his patient. True compassion can only come from struggling with and accepting one's own pain, limitations, failures, and conflicting motives.

The cultivation of self-acceptance also plays a central role in allowing therapists to acknowledge their contributions to the interaction and to disembed themselves from the patient's relational matrix. If therapists have difficulty becoming aware of and acknowledging feelings of anger, they will have difficulty unhooking themselves from vicious cycles that elicit anger. If they have difficulty acknowledging sexual feelings, then they will have difficulty disembedding from relational matrices in which sexual feelings play a role. The cultivation of self-acceptance by therapists play a critical role in helping them deal with inevitable impasses in the treatment. To the extent that their self-worth depends on having their patients change, they will have difficulty accepting the ways that they are stuck, and this will interfere with their ability to see new developments emerging that can provide a way out of the impasse.

Understanding Alliance Ruptures and Therapeutic Impasses

This chapter presents a variety of complementary lenses through which one can view therapeutic impasses. Each section highlights a different dimension relevant to understanding the processes through which ruptures in the therapeutic alliance take place and are resolved. Some articulate broad theoretical perspectives that provide a useful context for thinking about therapeutic impasses and outline relevant theoretical debates in the literature. Others provide more specific models for understanding the relevant therapeutic change processes. The danger of any theory is that it can lead to reification, thereby standing between the therapist and the patient and detracting from the mutuality and authentically human quality of the encounter. On the other hand, if used lightly, theory can point the therapist toward the exploration of possibilities emerging within the evolving interactive matrix that might otherwise be missed (see Aron, 1998, 1999; Hoffman, 1994; Spezzano, 1998, for related discussions). As we see it, the task for therapists is to find a way of using existing theory for purposes of facilitating the process of reflection-in-action (Schon, 1983), rather than for purposes of structuring their thinking about the clinical situation. In other words, theory can provide the therapist with leads, but the therapist's real task is to engage in a dialogue with the ever-changing clinical situation, through which existing theory is tested, fleshed out, and modified on an ongoing basis. This is particularly critical in the context of therapeutic impasses where therapists' anxiety can easily prompt them to lock into existing theoretical ideas.

HOPE AND DESPAIR

The problem of faith lies at the heart of the human change process. Despite Freud's best efforts to distance psychoanalysis from it roots in hypnosis and suggestibility, faith inevitably plays a role in any healing process. Whether one seeks relief from physical or emotional pain in the form of medication, spirituality, or psychotherapy, at some fundamental level one must believe that things can be different. One has to have some confidence that one has the ability to change and some hope that the healer has the ability to help one change. All people in psychotherapy struggle with varying degrees of demoralization. In many cases the balance between hope and despair is such that the patient can readily come to believe in the therapist's good will and potency and in the value of the therapeutic process. In some cases, however, the process of developing faith is a struggle of Herculean proportions. When one's life experience has been such that one has little faith that others will be willing or able to act on one's behalf, the process of cultivating such hope becomes *the* problem of psychotherapy. In many cases, the severity of patients' bitterness, cynicism, and despair makes it virtually impossible for them to find any kind of solace or comfort from another human being and leaves others thwarted in their efforts to make contact with them or be helpful to them. Such cases are likely to engender intense countertransference feelings in the therapist.

Often people hide the full intensity of their despair from others because of their belief that others will be alienated by it. They also hide the full intensity of their despair from themselves because it feels too painful to fully acknowledge. When one feels hopeless, the first step in the process of cultivating faith involves fully acknowledging and owning one's despair and sharing it with another human being. Consequently, therapists must be vigilant for any indication of cynicism or despair in patients when they first begin therapy. The therapist's task is to encourage the patient to bring whatever cynicism, anger, or despair that he or she is feeling into the here-and-now of the therapeutic relationship. In this way, a vague, generalized feeling of hopelessness and despair that the patient experiences in isolation can be transformed into a concrete feeling of hopelessness in a specific relational context.

This transformation accomplishes a number of things. First, by articulating his feelings of hopelessness to the therapist, the patient acknowledges these feelings more fully to himself. This process helps the patient to contact the pain underlying the feeling of having given up and reactivates the unfulfilled yearning, which the patient may not be fully in contact with. This yearning provides an opening for human contact. Second, by articulating these feelings to the therapist, the patient begins to feel less isolated. The patient thus begins the journey back from exile to being a member of the human community. If the therapist is able to respond to the patient's despair without shrinking or withdrawing, the patient begins to see that he does not have to be alone in his despair. By responding to the patient's despair in a compassionate and understanding fashion, the therapist provides the patient with the experience of being cared for and connected to another in his or her pain.

> Benjamin was a 36-year-old man who was extremely socially isolated and had never had a long-term relationship with a woman. Although Benjamin acknowledged being distressed by his circumstances, the therapist was surprised by the relative degree of equanimity with which he appeared to be dealing with the situation. He had initially been referred by a relative, approximately a year prior to beginning treatment, but maintained that he had not contacted the therapist at that time because he didn't feel that his problems were severe enough to warrant treatment. He had no previous treatment experience and knew nothing about therapy. On the face of things, Benjamin was optimistic about the possibility of being helped and open to giving things a try. From the outset, however, the therapist had an intuitive sense of a subtle element of cynicism in Benjamin's attitudes about treatment and about life in general; this cynicism was revealed as much in the way he spoke as in the specifics of what he said. The therapist also became aware of a growing feeling on his own part of inadequacy, a sense that somehow nothing he could do would be helpful to Benjamin. Although it was difficult for the therapist to articulate what aspects of Benjamin's presentation, if any, evoked these feelings in him, he consistently experienced himself at a loss to say anything that he imagined might be meaningful to Benjamin. His understanding, in retrospect, was that Benjamin's difficulty in acknowledging his feelings of despair had left him affectively frozen and unavailable and that the subtle hints of cynicism that the therapist had been picking up were the only threads linking to Benjamin's underlying longing and vitality.
>
> A good deal of the work in the first phase of treatment involved the therapist giving feedback regarding his intuitions about Benjamin's cynicism and his own feelings of impotence vis-à-vis

him, and helping Benjamin to acknowledge and articulate this cynicism. For example, in one session in which the therapist was feeling particularly stymied, he said to Benjamin, "I've been feeling something for some time, and I'm not sure what it means, but I feel at a loss to say anything that might be helpful to you. Somehow I imagine nothing I might say will seem meaningful to you." In his response, Benjamin was able to acknowledge that it was difficult for him to imagine the therapist saying anything helpful or meaningful. The therapist responded, "It sounds to me like you're feeling kind of cynical and not too hopeful about things between us." In turn, Benjamin was able to begin acknowledging these feelings and with the therapist's encouragement was able to begin elaborating about them. Over time, his initial tentative acknowledgment of an edge of cynicism deepened into an exploration of deep and corrosive feelings of bitterness and hopelessness. Gradually, Benjamin was able to become more frank with the therapist about his skepticism concerning the therapist's ability to help him and his suspiciousness of the therapist's motives for treating him. He confessed to suspecting that the therapist had no faith in the possibility of helping him and that the therapist was just meeting with him as a way to make money. Over time, the therapist's growing ability to listen to Benjamin's skepticism about his competence and motivation in a nondefensive fashion helped Benjamin to become a little less mistrustful, and to deepen his exploration of his feelings of helplessness and despair. As Benjamin was able to contact and articulate these feelings, the therapist began to feel less paralyzed and to develop more of a sense of affective engagement with Benjamin. In turn, Benjamin began to experience his own pain more deeply, and the therapist's feelings of empathic connection to Benjamin deepened.

In the first phase of treatment an important focus of the therapist's internal work involved observing his instinctive tendency to distance himself from Benjamin with feelings of anger, condescension, or dismissiveness and then tracking the flow of inner experience back to his own underlying feelings of impotence, futility, and despair. Over time, the process of fully acknowledging these feelings to himself and dwelling on them and associated memories began to reopen internal space that had been collapsed by his own need to defend against them. In this type of internal work, it is important to open oneself to pockets of despair in one's own life, both past and present. Theodore Jacobs's (1991) approach to countertransference exploration is particularly relevant here.

When the therapist was growing up, his sister had been chronically depressed, and his role was to make her happy. The periodic moments of success that he experienced were rewarding, but he also came to resent this responsibility, as well as his sister's

failure to help herself. During one session with Benjamin, he recalled a memory of a telephone conversation with his sister that
had taken place 10 years earlier when he was in his early 30s. During the conversation, he had been exasperated with her apparent
helplessness and inability to do anything to change her life situation. His sister had sensed his exasperation and said to him, "You
don't understand. I don't have any will." Perhaps he had been able
to hear her in a new way because of changes that were already taking place in him. Perhaps it was his sister's intuiting of these
changes that let her say what she said. In retrospect, the event, in
the therapist's mind, had marked a turning point in his relationship to his sister's despair, as well as to his own.

In the years following this incident with his sister, a number of
events in his own life had led the therapist to confront his own feelings of despair more deeply, and he had simultaneously come to
experience less of a need to help her and less of a tendency to
judge her harshly for her inability to change. As he worked with
Benjamin, the therapist recalled some of these difficult episodes
in his own life, when it had felt impossible to communicate the
depths of his despair to anyone else, when he could not imagine
the painful feelings ending, and when the prospect of someone
else being there for him in a meaningful way seemed inconceiv-
able. He also dwelled on areas in his current life where he felt
stuck and at times hopeless—ways in which the same conflicts he
remembered struggling with in his early adulthood continued to
play themselves out with dreary monotony. This process helped to
rekindle a feeling of compassion for himself in his own struggles
and his impotence with Benjamin. This in turn helped him feel
more accepting of Benjamin.

Gradually, treatment moved into a phase in which isolated
moments of hopefulness began to emerge for Benjamin. These
would typically take place following an extended interaction between patient and therapist during which the therapist had helped
Benjamin to articulate whatever cynical feelings he had about his
therapist and the therapy, without responding defensively. What
was striking, however, was that these moments of hopefulness
would immediately be followed by Benjamin's return to his more
customary state of cynicism and hopelessness. This shift would
take place so quickly that the therapist would be unaware of it until
he would find himself locked into a futile attempt to reassure
Benjamin or to convince him that things would get better. When
he was able to track these rapid shifts in Benjamin's self-states as
they took place and explore his experience in the moment,
Benjamin was able to articulate a fear of being "conned" or "taken
in" by the therapist. This, it emerged, would lead him to retreat to
his familiar self-protective, cynical stance. Over time, this fear of

being conned became further fleshed out into a concern that any feelings of hope would inevitably lead to disappointment and more pain. Gradually, the process of articulating his fear of hoping, both to himself and to the therapist, helped Benjamin to sustain longer and longer periods of trust, both in their relationship and in the therapy process. They then began to move into a new phase of the treatment in which the moments of hope became less isolated and Benjamin's predominant experience of despair began to give way to an underlying longing for nurturance and support.

RESISTANCE: INTRAPSYCHIC, CHARACTEROLOGICAL, AND RELATIONAL

In classical psychoanalytic theory, therapeutic impasses were often understood to stem from the patient's resistance. Over the years, the psychoanalytic literature on resistance has evidenced a number of significant shifts in perspective. Traditionally, *resistance* has been understood as any aspect of the patient's activity (either intrapersonal or interpersonal) that obstructs the therapeutic process. As Greenson (1967) put it, "Resistance means opposition. [It is] all those forces within the patient which oppose the procedures and the processes of analysis" (p. 60). There is an ambivalent relationship to the concept of resistance in psychoanalytic theory. On the one hand, many theorists recognize that the analysis of resistance lies at the heart of the therapeutic process and that this process *is* the therapy, rather than something that paves the way for the therapy. On the other hand, there is the persistent notion that although the analysis of resistance is central, the ultimate goal of therapy is to get at the impulse that is defended against.

In the early days of psychoanalysis the goal was to get at repressed memories and affect. Over time, there was an important shift in the direction of recognizing the importance of understanding or analyzing the resistances, rather than bypassing them. The development of Freud's (1923) structural theory was an important step in this process. Prior to the development of structural theory, anxiety was viewed as a by-product of dammed-up psychic energy. It was believed that bringing unconscious material into awareness would free up this energy and eliminate the anxiety. Resistance was viewed as a barrier to be bypassed or overcome. With the development of structural theory, Freud began to see anxiety as a signal of the potential breakthrough of dangerous instinctual impulses. Resistance was now seen as the ego's response to the perceived danger of being overwhelmed. This paved the way for a technical approach that involves attempting to explore and understand this perception of danger.

Wilhelm Reich's (1949) work on character analysis was another important step in the development of the perspective that resistance needs to be understood. Reich argued for the importance of viewing defensive processes holistically as part of the individual's overall way of being-in-the-world rather than as isolated mechanisms of defense. He advocated going beyond a microscopic approach to wish/defense analysis toward a more holistic approach to analyzing the individual's entire character structure. This structure consists of attitudes, beliefs, values, wishes, fantasies, ambitions, and other aspects of the individual's overall personality. Thus character structure consists of an overall style of living that provides protection against psychic danger. The value of Reich's approach is that it recognizes that resistances are more than forces that oppose therapeutic progress. They constitute an important part of the individual's character. From this perspective, the analysis of resistance provides the therapist with important information about the patient's fundamental way of being-in-the-world.

There are, however, shortcomings to Reich's perspective. Despite his recognition that defenses constitute an intrinsic part of one's character, his perspective has a tendency to view one's character structure as merely defensive. This tendency is linked to his romanticization of the instinctual. Moreover, character analysis, if insensitively applied, can harm the therapeutic alliance. For example, the therapist who is too eager to point out the defensive function of a patient's positive attitude toward him may undermine the rapport necessary for the working relationship. As Schafer (1983) notes,

> Reich himself shows in his militaristic metaphors of armor and attack how much one may fall into an adversarial view of the analytic relationship. Despite his rich understanding of the analysand's needing to resist and the complex meaning or function of this policy, he, like so many others, lapses into speaking of it as though it were a motiveless form of stubbornness or belligerence. (p. 73)

With the further development of ego psychology, a general understanding emerged that analysis should proceed from surface to depth. As Fenichel (1941) put it,

> Analysis must always go on in the layers accessible to the ego at the moment. When an interpretation has no effect, one often asks oneself, "How could I have interpreted more deeply?" But often the question should more correctly be put, "How could I have interpreted more superficially?" (p. 41)

A decade later, Ernst Kris (1951) continued in the same vein: "Resistance is no longer simply an 'obstacle' to analysis, but part of the psychic surface, which has to be explored" (p. 19). And yet there is still a residual tendency to regard the "surface" aspects of the patient's psyche as defensive and as less real than its deeper aspects. It has been difficult to completely move beyond the tendency to view resistances as obstacles that have to be ultimately overcome (Sandler, Dare, & Holder, 1992).

Paul Gray (1994) has referred to this tendency as a "developmental lag" between theory and technique. He and Fred Busch (1995) argue that there are probably a number of factors accounting for the persistent tendency to treat resistance as an obstacle despite this long-standing theoretical shift. These include the fact that (1) therapists cannot help but be fascinated by the search for hidden meaning, and this leads them to be more interested in what is being defended against, rather than the process of resistance itself; (2) the instinctive feeling that patients are trying to thwart us when resistance emerges, and the feelings of anger that emerge as a consequence; and (3) a desire to be in the position of the expert who is able to know what goes on for our patients unconsciously.

British object relations theorists have not emphasized the importance of resistance analysis to the same extent as ego analysts. Theorists such as Fairbairn (1952) and Guntrip (1969) have, however, attempted to develop a generally more affirmative stance toward resistance (see Aron, 1996). They conceptualized resistance as based on the fear of retraumatization, and as stemming from the patient's fears of appearing weak and inadequate. They emphasize the role that feelings of shame and humiliation play in motivating resistance. Similarly, Kohut (1971, 1977) viewed resistance as the attempt to avoid the repetition of traumatic experience. According to him, resistances are healthy and necessary functions of the self. They stem from the patient's experience of the treatment as dangerous. Thus it is critical for therapists to attempt to provide the conditions that will help the patient to feel safe and to acknowledge empathic failures on their part that may contribute to resistance.

Roy Schafer (1992) has also critiqued the persistent tendency to view resistance in pejorative terms and has emphasized that resistance is a part of the process, rather than an obstacle to it. He also maintains that what we tend to think of as resistance can be better understood as behaviors on the patient's part that elicit negative countertransference in therapists. Schafer emphasizes the importance of attempting to understand this negative countertransference, rather than thinking of the patient as resisting.

Another theoretical shift that has implications for the way we view resistance is the recent tendency to view the self as multiple and discontinuous (e.g., Bromberg, 1998; Mitchell, 1993; Pizer, 1998). Philip Bromberg (1996), for example, argues that while in reality there are multiple selves, there is a natural motivation to preserve the experience of self-continuity and that resistance often emerges when this experience is threatened (this perspective is compatible with the view held by constructivist cognitive therapists such as Giovanni Liotti, 1987; Vittorio Guidano, 1991; and Michael Mahoney, 1991). According to Bromberg (1995), resistance emerges when the intervention that the therapist offers is "experienced at that moment as requiring the patient to trade off some domain of his own self-experience for something he is being offered that is 'not me' and that the analyst's offering is being opposed, in one way or another, because it is not felt as sufficiently negotiable" (p. 176). From this perspective, what is traditionally conceptualized as resistance is seen as a part of the self that has an important function. It is no less real or important than other parts of the self (e.g., the self wishing to collaborate with the therapist on the current therapeutic task). Thus it is critical for the therapist to be able to ally and dialogue with this aspect of the self.

A final significant shift in the literature on resistance concerns its conceptualization from a two-person perspective. The concept of resistance originated in the context of a one-person psychological perspective. From this perspective, it is assumed that it is possible to understand an obstruction in the therapeutic process independent of the relational context in which it takes place. From a two-person psychological perspective, any apparent obstruction in the therapeutic process must be understood as a function of the interaction between the patient and the therapist. A patient's resistance may be an understandable response to the therapist's actions or attitudes (both conscious and unconscious) that are communicated at a subtle level. A patient who "resists" a particular interpretation of his motives may be responding in part to an implicit negative judgment on the therapist's part. A patient who has difficulty accessing painful emotional material is having difficulty accessing it in a specific relational context. This difficulty must be understood both intrapsychically and interpersonally.

The exploration of the resistance to acknowledging a specific emotion may lead to the elucidation of a generalized and unconscious belief the patient has that such feelings are dangerous. It is critical, however, for the therapist to move beyond the elucidation of such generalized attitudes about such emotions to the exploration of the patient's expectations of what will happen if such emotions are experienced or expressed in the here-and-now of the therapeutic relationship. In conducting this type of exploration, the therapist must be willing to explore his or her own contribution to the situation and to acknowledge both to himself or herself and to the patient that the patient's fears may in fact be based upon an accurate perception of some aspect of the therapist's actions or attitudes.

WILL AND RESPONSIBILITY

Although the topic of the will has been largely neglected by modern psychotherapy and psychology theorists, there are a few important exceptions (e.g., James, 1890; Farber, 1966; Mitchell, 1993; Shapiro, 1965, 1989). One of the most notable is Otto Rank (1945), who made the will a central focus of his later work. Rank argued that the role of the will should be one of the central concerns of modern psychology. He charted out in considerable detail the role that will plays in normal development, as well as the various ways in which things can go awry. For him, the ability to intentionally assert oneself within the world in a healthy fashion and to individuate from others involves the development of a healthy will.

Rank's concept of the development of the will is connected in an integral fashion to his conceptualization of the birth trauma. He saw the process of individuation from the mother as being an important and lifelong developmental task. According to Rank, the expression of will is first manifested in the form of what he referred to as "counterwill," that is, the assertion of will in opposition to the will of the other. He believed that the exertion of will is inherently guilt-producing because it involves individuation and separation from the parents. It is thus particularly likely to be suppressed or prevented from healthy development if one's parents have difficulty accepting one's initial acts of self-assertion and individuation.

For Rank, the development of a healthy will plays a central role in psychotherapy. In his thinking, the expression of the will is inextricably bound to the creative act, which for him was the sine qua non of healthy human existence and self-expression. Conversely, neurosis is typically associated with a paralysis of the will, resulting from the failure to achieve the important developmental task of achieving a sense of agency. According to him, therapy in some ways involves a recapitulation of the normal developmental process, and thus it is inevitable that patients will respond to therapists with counterwill in the same way that they did with their parents. Counterwill in therapy is expressed in the form of resistance. For Rank, resistance was not something to be overcome, worked through, or analyzed, but instead a process that should be nurtured, for it bears within it the seeds of healthy will. He believed that these seeds, if properly cultivated, will lead to the process of individuation and the creative expression of the self.

Rank's emphasis on the will stands in stark contrast to the prevailing silence on the topic in general psychoanalytic theory. It is worth inquiring into the reasons for this silence. Freud's emphasis on unconscious processes removed psychopathology from the moral realm. The essence of his perspective on psychic determinism was that people are motivated by instinctual forces outside of their own awareness. In Freud's view, psychological problems are to be understood as resulting from conflicts between instinct and the necessary evils of civilization, rather than as sinful acts resulting from failures of will. In this respect, he was challenging the Victorian notion of man as master of his own house and its emphasis on the primacy of willpower.

From an existential perspective, this view of psychic determinism is guilty of ignoring the importance of personal responsibility and intentionally in life. Jean-Paul Sartre (1943), for example, critiqued Freud's concept of the unconscious by arguing that it is a mechanistic metaphor that absolves the individual of personal responsibility and encourages a type of bad faith. Thus Sartre emphasized that the ego, which defends against unacceptable impulses, is ultimately nothing other than a part of the individual whose impulses are being defended against; the individual who disavows an impulse is ultimately divided against himself.

As Hellmuth Kaiser (1965) recognized, the neurotic is a person who is not "at one with his actions." In other words, he fails to take responsibility for his actions. More recently, Roy Schafer (1983) argued for replacing drive metatheory with what he refers to as "action language." In this framework, a repressed feeling is conceptualized as what he refers to as a "disclaimed action," that is, an action for which the actor accepts no responsibility.

The concept of responsibility, however, can be a double-edged sword. As therapists, it is inevitable that we will feel frustrated when our patients are not changing, and the line between understanding that our patients are ultimately responsible for their lives and defensively blaming them can sometimes by a fine one. As Kaiser (1965) argued, however, the patient's task is not to take responsibility for changing, but to experience responsibility for his or her own actions. The first step in taking responsibility for one's actions involves standing behind one's current actions, that is, experiencing one's current actions as chosen or willed. In order for one to do this, he or she must feel sufficiently self-accepting in the moment in the context of the relationship with the therapist. The fact that one is currently feeling self-critical prevents one from fully seeing the way in which one is currently choosing to live one's life in a self-defeating way. To experience oneself as choosing one's unfortunate life is a painful thing. A person in pain and distress is already full of self-loathing. He is feeling blamed for something over which he feels he has no control. It thus becomes extremely hard for him to acknowledge the way in which he may be contributing to his own problems. He has a constant experience of trying and yet failing and then feeling condemned by self and others for his failure. He thus experiences the will as atrophied. He has no experience of choosing his actions. An important element in the process of developing a sense of agency thus involves beginning to experience a sense of compassion for oneself. For this reason, the therapist who unconsciously feels condemning toward those who are not experiencing a sense of agency can make it even more difficult for them to begin to have such an experience. It is thus vital for us to be able to appreciate the phenomenological reality of being unable to will.

It is also helpful to remember that choices are not made at a global level, but rather on a moment-by-moment basis. Thus, in order for patients to begin to recover a sense of agency, it is helpful for them to discover the choices they are making in the moment in the therapeutic relationship. For example, the act of unconsciously resisting the exploration of a particular feeling or fantasy can be transformed into the act of intentionally deciding not to do so in the present moment.

One of the better opportunities for helping patients to begin to take responsibility for their actions is to help them begin to stand behind their actions in the therapeutic relationship. For example, the patient who has difficulty accessing painful or frightening feelings can be encouraged to experiment with saying, "I'm not willing to explore these feelings right now," rather than saying, "I don't know what I'm feeling." The therapist can then ask the patient what it feels like to make a statement of this type, or alternatively ask her to describe the nature of her reluctance to proceeding further. With interventions of this type, it is critical for the therapist to convey both explicitly and implicitly that the patient's decision not to engage in a certain therapeutic task will be respected as valid and legitimate.

As patients begin to develop a sense of their own ability to set limits with the therapist, they gain an increased sense of agency and ability to do something in opposition to the therapist directly, rather than indirectly. What was previously an unconscious defensive activity is transformed into a direct act of self-assertion. This type of acceptance of responsibility assumes therapeutic priority over an attempt to explore the experience that is being defended against. A patient who has ambivalent feelings about being in therapy may be encouraged to explore both sides of the ambivalence fully. A decision to leave therapy as a result of this type of exploration may be a better therapeutic outcome than continuing in therapy in a half-hearted way.

> In the early phases of treatment with Benjamin, he customarily talked about his daily experience in a very general and superficial fashion that omitted details of interactions, as well as any reference to underlying feelings or conflicts. Sessions often had a monotonous and redundant quality to them, with little, if any, sense of movement. When his therapist would give him feedback about his style and ask him if he had any awareness of it, he would respond that there was nothing important to talk about. In this context, his therapist would respond with a simple question such as "Do you have any awareness of choosing not to talk about something right now?" or "Are you aware of avoiding anything in this moment?" Although at first Benjamin did not indicate any such awareness, over time he was able to begin acknowledging some awareness of not wanting to touch on painful feelings of shame and humiliation. He would then condemn himself for cowardice and question the value of their work together, given that he felt unable to go into things more deeply. At this point, his therapist would emphasize that it was important for them to respect his need for privacy and for him not to push himself to talk about things before he was ready. This helped him to experience his resistance as legitimate and to stand behind it, rather than to experience it as something outside of his control.

Working in this way is reminiscent of Paul Gray's (1994) close process analysis. The emphasis, however, is on helping patients to experience the capacity to choose through identifying with a dissociated aspect of the self that is experienced to be in opposition to the therapist (Bromberg, 1995). Often with patients who feel completely stuck in their lives and have no capacity to choose and to act in accordance with their choices, the ability to will in opposition to the therapist can be a critical turning point in therapy. It is thus particularly important to be vigilant for subtle indications of nonresponsiveness, withdrawal, irritability, or criticism in patients, since (if properly explored) such indications can provide an opportunity for them to begin to express their counterwill in a more direct fashion.

> In Benjamin's case, some of the most powerful sessions were those in which he was able to explicitly criticize his therapist for not being more helpful to him. Early in treatment there were sessions in which the therapist felt that anything he said evoked a type of cold, sullen withdrawal on Benjamin's part and what felt like a pained

tolerance of his presence. On such occasions, the therapist would say something such as "It feels to me like the things I'm saying are really rubbing you the wrong way." In response, Benjamin would begin to acknowledge his anger at the therapist for not being of greater help to him. This was a difficult thing for him to express, for he felt that blaming the therapist was a reflection of his own immaturity. Over time, the therapist explored Benjamin's feelings of shame about his anger at the therapist, as well as his fear that the therapist would respond to his anger by abandoning him. The therapist showed a genuine interest in hearing about his anger. As he gradually came to express it more directly, Benjamin began to feel more empowered in his life in general.

IMPASSES AS WINDOWS INTO CORE ORGANIZING PRINCIPLES

Another important conceptual shift involves viewing therapeutic impasses as windows into the patient's relational schemas, rather than as obstacles to be overcome. This type of shift is particularly well represented in the writings of Robert Stolorow and colleagues (Stolorow et al., 1994), as well as in the work of contemporary Kleinians, such as Betty Joseph (1989). For Stolorow and colleagues, therapeutic impasses are the "royal road to analytic understanding." Building upon Heinz Kohut's (1984) emphasis on the central role that working through empathic failures plays in the change process, they emphasize the idea that the patient's experience of the therapist's interventions will inevitably be shaped by his or her core organizing principles (both conscious and unconscious). They are particularly interested in situations in which the therapist fails to adequately understand and respond t/ the patient's needs because of an intersection between the patient's a/ the therapist's core organizing principles. To provide one exam/ from Stolorow and Atwood (1992):

A female patient presents a seductive and coquettish style
motivated by a desperate need to be recognized and to co/
feelings of emptiness and worthlessness. The origins of t/
tive style can be traced back to her relationship with a se/
ther whose sexual attention provided the only excer
otherwise unconfirming and unresponsive family e
Her therapist, who is practicing in accordance w/
standing of the precepts of classical psychoanalysi
her urgent requests for affirming and mirroring r
be met either with silence or, at most, with bri/
The patient experiences the therapist's lack of '

repetition of the traumatically depriving circumstances of her childhood. She responds by alternating between escalations of her seductiveness and expressions of rage. Although the therapist's response to the patient can be understood, in part, in terms of his conceptual understanding of the principles of the therapeutic approach he is trying to apply, it can also be understood in terms of his own relational schema. He assimilates the patient's desperate demands for mirroring responsiveness into a preexisting sensitivity to the issues of power, control, and autonomy that derives from his own developmental experiences. These involved a relationship with an overly domineering mother, whom he experienced as tyrannical and oppressive and habitually responded to with stubborn resistance and withdrawal.

In this situation, a detailed exploration of both the patient's experience of the therapist's response and of the therapist's contribution to the interaction might potentially have transformed an impasse into a comprehensive understanding (which might otherwise be impossible to obtain) of the patient's relational schema. Formulations based upon the patient's narratives about past or present events are at best crude hypotheses. In contrast, therapeutic impasses provide an opportunity to investigate the subtle nuances of the patient's characteristic style of construing and acting as it unfolds in the present. When things are proceeding smoothly in therapy, it is paradoxically easy to "get by" without questioning the accuracy of our understanding of our patient's inner worlds or examining the way in which our own preconceptions or core organizing principles shape our understanding of our patients. Paradoxically, periods of impasse force us to deepen our understanding of our patients and to investigate our own contribution to the interaction. As Stolorow and colleagues highlight, it is impossible to understand patients without understanding the therapist's contribution to the interaction. As Renik (1993) puts it, "Every aspect of an analyst's clinical activity is determined in part by his or her personal psychology" (p. 553). Whether the therapist empathizes, interprets, confronts, challenges, or validates is always in part a reflection of the therapist's own personal dynamics. There is thus an irreducible subjectivity to everything the therapist says and does (Aron, 1996; Hoffman, 1998).

A further dimension on the role of impasses as windows into deeper understanding is pointed to by contemporary Kleinians such as Betty Joseph (1989). Joseph focuses on the importance of carefully tracking the patient's responsiveness to the therapist's interventions, since failure to make use of the therapist's interventions can reflect an important dynamic underlying the patient's general style of functioning. For example:

Joseph (1989, p. 199) describes a patient who is nearing termination and begins a session by discussing his anxiety about various events that are taking place in his life (e.g., he and his wife are in the process of selling their house). Joseph interprets the anxiety as being related to his imminent termination. The patient agrees, but then continues to discuss his generalized discomfort, and Joseph senses anger and resentment. She makes a second interpretation, suggesting that he has difficulty accepting the fact that she will let him leave treatment, because he thinks of himself as being a "very special patient" to her. The patient responds by continuing to discuss his difficulties in general, and again conveys a sense of resentment. At this point, Joseph interprets his anger and misery as a defense against dealing with painful feelings about termination. The patient becomes silent and then acknowledges that he has the thought: "clever old bag." Further exploration reveals he believes that Joseph is right, but feels envious and rivalrous because of this. Thus, careful tracking and exploration of the patient's moment-by-moment responses to interpretations, helps him to see the way in which his envy interferes with his ability to make use of them. He is then able to experience a less ambivalent appreciation of Joseph's insight and to contact feelings of sadness about termination.

What is particularly valuable about Joseph's contribution on this matter is her detailed attention to the microscopic aspects of patient and therapist interactions, as well as her focus on the potential role of the therapist's countertransference feelings in helping to illuminate what is going on in these interactions. Joseph's work highlights the importance of going beyond a focus on the type of intense or global impasses that are obvious to both patient and therapist, toward an investigation of the sometimes subtle ways in which patients deflect or neutralize the therapist's interventions. For example, a patient may agree with a therapist's interpretation, but the therapist will nevertheless be left with a subtle feeling that there is something funny about the patient's response. In situations of this type, the therapist's feelings provide a potential clue to aspects of the patient's dynamics that lead him or her to respond to interventions in a particular way.

From our perspective, however, Joseph's work (despite its virtues) fails to accord sufficient attention to the therapist's potential contribution to these subtle events. She also has a tendency to assimilate her understanding of the patient's intrapsychic processes into a preexisting formulation rather than to engage in a process of sustained empathic inquiry, which allows the patient's experience to reveal itself in its own terms. Nevertheless, there is something extremely important about her disciplined and intensive focus on the more molecular aspects of the patient's responsiveness (or lack thereof) to the therapist's interventions.

RESTRUCTURING THE PATIENT'S
RELATIONAL SCHEMAS

Like many recent innovations in contemporary psychoanalytic theory, the idea that working through a therapeutic impasse or a rupture in the therapeutic alliance in a constructive fashion can bring about or facilitate a restructuring of the patient's relational schemas can be traced back to Sandor Ferenczi (1932). He was the first to emphasize the idea that therapy often involves a reenactment of the patient's traumatic developmental experience in which the therapist is gradually pulled into playing the role of the perpetrator. From his perspective, a critical part of the change process involves the therapist recognizing his or her contribution to the interaction and then acknowledging it to the patient, thereby providing a new experience for the patient. As various authors have documented (e.g., Haynal, 1989; Aron & Harris, 1991; Wallerstein, 1995), Ferenczi's emphasis on the importance of the therapeutic relationship as a mechanism of change influenced a variety of theorists on both sides of the Atlantic, both directly and indirectly, but in many ways his contribution was marginalized until recent years.

In the 1940s and 1950s, Franz Alexander's (1948) notion of the corrective emotional experience emerged as a controversial challenge to the predominant emphasis on insight as the mechanism of change in mainstream psychoanalysis. In a manner clearly reminiscent of Ferenczi, Alexander argued that change takes place when the therapist is able to assume an attitude different than that which was assumed by the patient's parent in the original conflict situation. Alexander's position became the focus of a heated theoretical debate, with critics charging that he was employing suggestion rather than being truly analytic, that he was advocating that the therapist "play a role" (thereby being manipulative), and that his technical recommendations were based on the dubious assumption that the therapist would be able to correctly infer what type of role to play. While Alexander had a considerable following, over time the majority within the psychoanalytic community sided with his critics, and to this day Alexander's concept of the corrective emotional experience remains anathema to many.

Although Joseph Weiss (1993) is careful to distinguish between Alexander's position and his own, his control–mastery theory can in certain respects be seen as a contemporary version of the corrective emotional experience. Weiss, Harold Sampson, and their colleagues (1986) theorize that neurosis is the result of unconscious pathogenic beliefs that develop because of interactions with one's parents and other significant figures. These beliefs are inferred from experiences in childhood that were traumatizing to varying degrees. For example, a child whose father dies during his adolescence infers that acts of independence will destroy the other and thereafter renounces self-assertive striving. Examples of such pathogenic beliefs include the belief that acts of independence will lead to annihilation of the other, the belief that dependency will lead to abandonment, and the belief that anger will lead to retaliation. From the perspective of Weiss and colleagues (1986), the therapist's ability to act in a way that disconfirms the patient's perspective constitutes a central mechanism of change. For example, the therapist who does not retaliate in response to her patient's anger may disconfirm his pathogenic belief that aggression is dangerous. A therapist who does not become defensive when his patient speaks about terminating therapy may disconfirm his patient's belief that independence will be punished.

Control–mastery theory suggests two different ways in which a patient's pathogenic beliefs can be implicated in a therapeutic impasse or alliance rupture. In the first, the therapist may unwittingly act in a way that confirms the patient's pathogenic beliefs. For example, a patient believes that feelings of sadness will result in abandonment. The therapist fails to recognize how central a concern this is for the patient and consequently fails to adequately empathize with his sad feelings when they emerge. As a result, the patient cancels the next session. In this situation, only by coming to understand the meaning of her actions to the patient and empathizing with the patient's distress can the therapist refine her understanding of the patient's pathogenic belief and begin to disconfirm it.

In the second, a therapeutic impasse may be understood to be a manifestation of what Weiss et al. refer to as a "transference test." Weiss and colleagues (1986) theorize that people are motivated to act in a way that will test and hopefully disconfirm these beliefs, and that they are always unconsciously testing whether it is safe to acknowledge feelings, thoughts, and memories that have previously been warded off because of pathogenic beliefs. This process of testing pathogenic beliefs takes place both in everyday life and in the relationship with the therapist. For example, a patient who unconsciously believes that others will be hurt by acts of self-assertion may test this belief in the therapy by disagreeing with the therapist. If the therapist passes early transference tests by not becoming defensive when the patient disagrees, the patient may unconsciously decide that it is safe to engage in more substantial transference tests and thereafter may directly express anger at the therapist.

> A patient who unconsciously believed that she would be abandoned by other people if she depended on them began therapy by acting in a counterdependent fashion. As she became more trusting of the therapist, she began to express her anger at the therapist for not providing her with the support and direction she had hoped for. After an extended period of time during which the therapist responded in an understanding and nondefensive fashion, she began to acknowledge and express underlying feelings of sadness and pain about being emotionally isolated. When the therapist was able to respond in an empathic fashion, she was able to have the experience of feeling nurtured and cared for, a feeling that was new for her. Thus, a prolonged period in therapy that might be construed as an impasse was actually an important transference test.

Although control–mastery theory can provide a useful perspective on therapeutic impasses, one limitation is that it tends to assume that the therapist is sufficiently disembedded from the patient's relational matrix to develop an accurate formulation of the patient's pathogenic belief. As we have argued, the therapist will inevitably be embedded within the patient's relational matrix. Moreover, it is this very experience of being embedded in the patient's relational matrix that allows the therapist to come to some understanding of the patient's core relational schemas. Thus, from a relational perspective, therapeutic impasses often reflect the enactment of a relational pattern that in some respect parallels the patient's characteristic patterns, and it is the process of working one's way out of this embeddedness that restructures the patient's relational schemas.

AFFECTIVE MISCOORDINATION AND REPAIR

Recent research on affective communication in infant–mother interactions provides some intriguing suggestions regarding the role that emotional attunement and its absence may play in the developmental process, and by implication in the process of working through therapeutic impasses. As theory and research in the areas of emotion and infant development suggest, affective experience plays a central role in providing the individual with information about his or her own action dispositions (Greenberg & Safran, 1987; Lang, 1983; Leventhal, 1984).

The extent to which an individual integrates and synthesizes affective information of various types thus determines the extent to which he or she ultimately develops a sense of self that is grounded in his or her organismic, biologically rooted experience (Safran & Greenberg, 1991; Safran & Segal, 1990). Thus, as Daniel Stern (1985) points out, the process of affect attunement plays a central role in helping children to learn to experience and articulate a full range of emotions. Through this process, they develop a sense of self that is grounded in their own bodily-felt experience and that is communicable to the other.

A number of studies have demonstrated consistent differences between the way in which healthy and dysfunctional mother–infant dyads deal with moments of affective attunement and misattunement (Tronick, 1989). In both healthy and dysfunctional dyads, there is an ongoing oscillation between periods in which mother and infant are affectively attuned, or coordinated, and periods in which they are miscoordinated. In a healthy mother–infant dyad, moments of affective miscoordination are typically followed by a repair in the interaction. For example, a child begins to experience sadness or joy, and the mother misattunes to this emotion. In response to this misattunement, the child experiences a secondary emotion, such as anger. The mother then attunes to the secondary emotion, and the dyad becomes affectively coordinated once again. In contrast, in a dysfunctional mother–infant dyad, the mother not only fails to attune to the primary emotion, she also fails to attune to the secondary emotion.

Edward Tronick (1989), using Bowlby's model of internalization, suggests that in a healthy mother–infant dyad, the ongoing oscillation between periods of miscoordination and periods of repair ultimately serves a useful function by helping the infant to develop an adaptive relational schema, that is, one that represents the other as potentially available and the self as capable of negotiating relatedness even in the face of interactional rupture. In contrast, the infant in the dysfunctional dyad never develops this type of self–other representation, and as a result is likely to give up on the possibility of establishing authentic emotional contact. He or she does not develop faith in his or her ability to maintain authentic contact in the face of differences and in a desperate attempt to maintain some type of interpersonal relatedness will develop self-manipulative and other-manipulative strategies to maintain some type of interpersonal contact.

In the same way that the process of oscillating back and forth between states of affective miscoordination and repair is hypothesized to play a role in helping the infant to develop an adaptive relational schema, working through alliance ruptures may do so for the patient in psychotherapy. This process can provide a learning experience through which the patient gradually develops a relational schema that represents the other as potentially available and the self as capable of negotiating relatedness even in the context of interactional ruptures (Safran, 1993a; Safran & Segal, 1990).

RECOVERING A SPLIT-OFF PART OF THE SELF

A number of theorists have conceptualized the process of working through therapeutic impasses as playing a role in helping patients to recover a split-off part of the self. This theme can also be traced back to the early days of psychoanalysis in the writings of Sandor Ferenczi. Ferenczi (1931) suggested that neurosis develops as a result of splitting off a part of the self in order to maintain a relationship with one's parents. According to him, the infant, who is traumatized by his or her parents either sexually or emotionally, splits off part of the self and thereafter relates through a false self. This way of relating is designed to buy time until he can find a situation in which he can safely allow the split-off part of the self to reemerge. The child who splits off part of the self in this fashion experiences a paralysis of spontaneity and a kind of precocious maturity.

Extending this perspective, Winnicott (1956) maintained that when the infant is born, he or she is completely dependent upon the mother. By the same token, the mother is predisposed to be highly sensitive and very responsive to the infant's needs. At this point, she is in what Winnicott referred to as the "state of primary maternal preoccupation." According to him, the mother, by virtue of her sensitivity to the infant's needs, becomes sufficiently adapted to him or her to facilitate the omnipotent illusion that the mother and her need-fulfilling responses exist as a result of the infant's fantasy. By being attuned to the infant's needs in this fashion, the mother helps him integrate his spontaneous experience into his sense of self, thereby laying the foundation for the experience of feeling "real" and alive. This is the foundation of what Winnicott referred to as the "true self."

The *true self* is the source of authenticity in a person. It develops out of the mother's ability to provide what Winnicott called a "holding environment" for the infant, which meets his or her spontaneous expressions or gestures. When the mother fails to meet such gestures, the infant has to comply with her response in order to survive. The strategies of compliance that emerge are what Winnicott termed the "false self." The *false self* hides and protects the true self by complying with environmental demands. All human beings develop false selves, even under the most fortuitous circumstances. However, in extreme cases, when the mother repeatedly fails to recognize the infant's gestures and imposes her own responses on the infant, the true self is so hidden as to seem absent. The result is a pervasive sense of unreality, futility, and lack of vitality.

Ferenczi (1931) was the first to emphasize the importance of employing the therapeutic relationship to provide a "new beginning" for the patient (Balint's [1968] terminology): one in which he or she can learn to maintain a relationship with the analyst without the cost of splitting off part of the self. He spoke about the importance of using the analytic situation to allow the patient to abandon himself or herself to what he termed the phase of "passive object-love," that is, that phase in which, like the child, his or her needs are responded to perfectly by the other. Similarly, Winnicott believed in the importance of providing patients with a holding environment. He believed that with some patients it is important to promote the reemergence of dependency needs by facilitating a regression in the holding environment of the therapeutic relationship. This process allows the true self to emerge.

The idea of recovering a split-off part of the self has important implications for understanding therapeutic impasses. Misalliances often involve a type of false self compliance, which reflects the patient's characteristic way of relating to life. Such a false self misalliance inevitably involves an experience of hopelessness. By providing a holding environment for the patient and by empathizing with the totality of the patient's experience without being overwhelmed by it, the therapist can facilitate the emergence of true self experience; that is, the therapist can bring to the surface a buried well of authenticity and vitality.

While the notion that working through therapeutic impasses can help patients to recover a split-off part of the self can be heuristically valuable, it can also be problematic. The idea that there is a true self waiting to be discovered can encourage therapists to relate to other aspects of their patients as false or as merely defensive. Thus, for example, the analytical style of the intellectualized patient may be responded to by the therapist in a subtly critical and impatient fashion. The gentleness of the patient who is afraid of his own aggression may be regarded as exclusively defensive, rather than as a real feature of his character that has real value. Reifying the distinction between true and false selves can thus lead therapists to selectively value certain aspects of their patients' ways-of-being over others. This can make it more difficult for patients to become more fully accepting of themselves.

From the perspective of multiple selves discussed in Chapter 2, there is no unitary, static true self waiting to be discovered, but rather multiple self-states contending for dominance in awareness at any given moment. This perspective thus provides a useful corrective to a static and reified distinction between true and false selves. As previously indicated, Buddhist psychology provides an even more radical corrective. From this perspective, even the notion of multiple selves is a type of reification. It implies the presence of a finite number of substantial selves that can be known. Buddhist psychology, however, maintains that the self is an illusion that is constructed on a moment-by-moment basis. Change results from seeing through this illusion and surrendering to *being*.

Although Winnicott used the terminology of true versus false selves, his thinking on the issue was in many ways consistent with this type of perspective. In his writing, he alluded over and over again to a mode of being that involves simply *being*, rather than striving or doing. This capacity to be is associated with what he referred to as a "state of unintegration." He contrasted this state of unintegration to one of either ego integration or of ego disintegration. In his words, "The opposite of integration would seem to be disintegration. That is only partly true. The opposite, initially, requires a word like unintegration. Relaxation for an infant means not feeling a need to integrate, the mother's ego-supportive function being taken for granted" (Winnicott, 1965, p. 61). Thus, for Winnicott, this capacity *to be* is associated with a basic faith that the other will be there. It is also associated with a capacity to be alone, in the context of this basic trust that the other will be there when needed (Winnicott, 1958b).

TRANSITIONAL EXPERIENCE

The danger of becoming overly adapted to "objective reality" (i.e., reality as defined by others) is that one loses one's own sense of vitality and realness. Both Winnicott (1958a) and Kohut (1971) emphasized that it is developmentally critical for infants to experience an omnipotent or narcissistic stage in which others are sufficiently adapted to their needs in order for them to have the experience of being at the center of the world, before the process of disillusionment begins. Winnicott's concept of transitional space adds another important dimension to our understanding of the process of optimal disillusionment.

From his perspective, the process of healthy development does not involve a progressive relinquishment of illusion and a matching acceptance of reality, but rather a capacity to both accept reality and experience illusion. According to Winnicott, this capacity involves the ability to enter into the realm of what he referred to as "transitional space." *Transitional space* exists in an intermediate area between the realms of fantasy and reality, subjective and objective, or internal and external. Transitional experience (i.e., the ability to enter into this metaphorical space) involves the capacity to accept the paradox that something is simultaneously real and illusory. It thus serves as a bridge between inner and outer worlds and as an alternative to the mutually exclusive options of subjective or objective.

The prototypical transitional experience consists of the child's relationship to her favorite teddy bear or doll. In establishing a unique relationship with such an inanimate object, the child bestows special meaning on it, thereby making it more than just a teddy bear or doll. In a sense, it comes alive for the child, and in so doing provides her with emotional comfort and security. In this paradoxical situation the child bestows upon the bear or doll the very power it needs in order to be alive for the child in the way she needs it to be. But if children were to experience the transitional object as exclusively their own creation, it would no longer have the meaning they need it to have. Yet at some level they know that they have given it the meaning that it has. Transitional experience thus involves a type of "playing" in the sense that the boundaries between what is real and what is not real are temporarily blurred. It is also a form of playing in that it is a creative act through which one's internal experience is brought out into the world and in some sense made real.

Transitional experiencing is not merely a developmental interlude. It constitutes an important realm within healthy adult experience. In adult form, it is expressed as a capacity to play with one's fantasies, one's ideas, and the world's possibilities in a way that allows for the surprising and new to emerge. In order to experience transitional phenomena, one has to be able to experience one's internal world as meaningful, and this in turn requires a fundamental sense of trust in the other's willingness to be interested in one's internal world and responsive to one's emotional needs. Impasses in therapy often reflect the patient's inability to enter into a transitional space and the resulting sterility of his or her experience and inability to experience anything, including the therapeutic process, as meaningful. In such situations, words can become meaningless, and both life and the self can become emptied and deadened. In such situations, it is sometimes helpful for the therapist to be receptive to the development of a type of transitional experience through which he and his patients begin to work on important relational themes in "play" that they might not be able to work on more explicitly (see Newirth, 1995).

A session with Ashley, a patient described in Chapter 1, provides an illustration of this type of process. Recall that Ashley was a single young woman, who sought treatment because of a general sense of emptiness and meaninglessness in her life. She had suffered considerable emotional abuse and neglect from her parents and had developed a type of precocious maturity as a way of dealing with her unmet dependency needs. In the early phases of treatment, she had considerable difficulty exploring painful topics and feelings and rejected any attempts to talk about what was going on in the therapeutic relationship. Her general stance was one of mistrust and wariness. Many sessions were filled with superficial conversation, followed by long, angry silences. Ashley consistently complained that the treatment wasn't helping, and when asked what was missing, replied that she needed more guidance and direction. She also complained about the therapist's lack of self-disclosure. Feeling thwarted in his attempts to explore what was going on in the therapeutic relationship in greater depth, the therapist decided to experiment with providing more of the guidance and support that Ashley said was missing. He also began to experiment with being more intentionally self-revealing, hypothesizing that Ashley's request for more self-disclosure was a way of saying, "I'm not going to take the risk of opening up for you until you're willing to demonstrate that you're willing to invest in this relationship by risking more openness yourself." Over time, the quality of the relationship began to shift and she began to become somewhat more trusting and open.

Nevertheless, many sessions continued to begin with the superficial conversation followed by silence that was characteristic of treatment at the beginning. During one such silence, Ashley turned to a picture of the therapist's daughter that he kept in his office and asked if he had recently changed the picture in the frame. The therapist replied that the picture had not been changed since she began treatment, and asked her what she saw in the picture. She replied, "I see a child who looks like she's kind of sad and afraid. What do you see?" The therapist responded, "I see my daughter whom I love." At this point, Ashley began to cry. The therapist asked her what was going on for her, and she began to talk about the lack of nurturance and love in her own life.

The therapist's motivation for his actions, no doubt, had multiple determinants, some conscious and some not. At one level, he sensed that the picture was a projective and that Ashley was speaking about herself when she spoke about the emotions she attributed to the child in the picture. At another level, perhaps she was saying, "You're not a very good father, either to your daughter or to me." He also sensed that to try to address her feelings directly at this point or to attempt to interpret them would be rejected. Moreover, to fail to respond to Ashley's question would likely be experienced by her as withholding. At the same time, the therapist felt touched by the little girl side of Ashley that he sensed desperately wanted emotional nurturance even though she was unable to open herself to accept it. Talking about his love for his own daughter was perhaps, in part, an indirect way of expressing his caring for Ashley. Perhaps it was, in part, a way of saying, "I care about my daughter, in her sadness and fear, and I care about you as well." Perhaps part of it was also a way of dealing with his own feelings of sadness emerging through identification with Ashley's pain, by reaffirming for himself his feelings of loving connection with his own daughter. Perhaps there was even an angry or defensive element to his response. For example, "Despite what you may think, I really am a good father. I care about my daughter, and I'm willing to prove my ability to be a good father to you by responding to your wish to speak openly about my feelings, even if it highlights the absence of a similar loving connection in our relationship."

Similarly, it is impossible to definitively understand Ashley's response to the therapist's remarks. Perhaps at one level she experienced the therapist's remarks as an indirect expression of his empathy and caring for her. Perhaps at another level his expression of his love for his daughter accentuated her own sense of aloneness in reminding her of her parent's failures, as well as the fact that in real life the therapist could never be a loving father for her the way he was for his own daughter.

Interactions of this type are difficult to make sense of in any kind of definitive fashion. They defy linear, sequential understanding and instead have a type of intuitive resonance to them as they are happening. Although an attempt to make logical sense of them can be made in retrospect, it can at best provide a partial understanding. Although the therapist empathized with Ashley's feelings of sadness and explored her desire for love and nurturance in her life, he made no attempt in this session to sort out the precise meaning of their interaction. While in some situations this type of retrospective analysis can be helpful, in others it can be a way of diluting or undoing something genuine that has taken place in the relationship. As Hoffman (1998) points out, the compulsive need to analyze everything, itself needs to be analyzed. In this situation, Ashley's response suggested that the therapist's disclosure had facilitated the therapeutic process, and he felt that to explicitly explore the meaning of what had gone on in their relationship would be to take away with one hand (through emphasizing the nonmutuality of the relationship by resuming the role of the analyzing therapist) what he had given with the other (i.e., a willingness to emphasize the mutual aspect of the relationship through self-disclosure).

OPTIMAL DISILLUSIONMENT

In life, we all must inevitably deal with the fact that by the very nature of our existence we are simultaneously alone and at the same time cast into the world with others. We are alone at a fundamental level in that we are born alone and ultimately must die alone. Although we are able to share many things with other people, many of our private experiences will never be shared with them. At the same time, we are inescapably tied to others. We are born in relationship to others and attain a sense of self only in relation to others. As current developmental research makes increasingly clear, human beings are biologically programmed to seek relationships with other people and to develop in the context of relationships with other people. Yet despite the intrinsically interpersonal nature of human existence, we are ultimately encapsulated by our own skin and set apart from others by virtue of our existence as independent organisms. As human beings we thus spend our lives negotiating the paradox of our simultaneous aloneness and togetherness. We begin our lives attempting to remain in proximity to attachment figures, and the pursuit of interpersonal relatedness continues to motivate our behavior through our lifetimes. No matter how hard we try, however, we cannot, except for brief periods, achieve the type of union with others that permits us to escape from our aloneness.

Michael Balint (1968) coined the term the "basic fault" to describe the fundamental experience many people have that there is something wrong or missing. According to him, this *basic fault* arises from the experience of disruption of the archaic state of what he termed "primary object relation" or "primary love." He argued, as did Rank (1948), that the experience of birth is traumatic in that the infant is separated from the state of biological symbiosis with the mother, what he termed a "harmonious interpenetrating mix-up" (Balint, 1968). According to him, this primary experience of relatedness in the intrauterine environment is continued to some extent following birth, as the mother continues to cater to the infant's needs, in a fashion that the infant takes for granted. Inevitably, however, the mother falls short of complete and total responsiveness, and the infant experiences a disruption in this harmonious state. The basic fault is thus the experience of a mismatch or a discrepancy between the needs of the particular individual and the capacity of people in the environment to provide for them.

According to Jacques Lacan (1953, 1973b), we all exist in a fundamental state of alienation (or what he refers to as "lack"), in which we sense that something is missing. This is true for a number of reasons. First, there is the fact that we can only express ourselves through the distorting medium of language. Second, and relatedly, our existence as subjects is tied to the desire of the other. Our parents' desires become our own, and it is difficult if not impossible to completely disentangle them. Third, from the beginning, the child would like to be the sole object of his or her mother's affection, but the mother's desire always goes beyond the child (to the father, among others). There is thus a normal process of separation from the undifferentiated symbiotic union with the mother, mediated in part by the presence of the father or some symbolic equivalent (Lacan speaks about the "father's name" or the paternal function in order to make it clear that he is not necessarily referring to the actual father). Because of this split, people spend their lives pursuing experiences and relationships that are symbolic reminders of this lost unity in the unconscious hope of recapturing the experience of wholeness. By its very nature, however, this desire can never be fully satisfied.

This fundamental sense that there is something missing, of having fallen from a state of grace, is a universal theme in mythology, and the attempt to heal this basic fault is a central concern in all spiritual traditions. In Judeo-Christian tradition, this sense of having fallen from a state of grace is reflected in the myth of the expulsion from the Garden of Eden. Jewish culture is imbued with a sense of living in exile, both as a historical and as a cosmic principle. Both Jewish and Christian traditions are concerned with healing our sense of separateness through obtaining a sense of union with the divine and with fellow human beings. This is particularly true of the Kabbalistic and Hasidic traditions in Judaism and of the Gnostic traditions in Christianity. The Hindu tradition sees the dilemma of the experience of human separateness as arising from the failure to recognize that we are all part of one universal essence, Brahma, and the recognition and experience of our fundamental being as part of this universal essence, as the solution. Buddhism views the basic human dilemma as arising from a mistaken conception of self as having a permanent and substantial nature and from the recognition of the nonduality of self and others as the solution.

A recurring theme in the literature is that working through therapeutic impasses involves a type of optimal disillusionment. As Winnicott (1956) suggested, the mother's absolute attunement to the infant cannot last forever. Gradually, as she moves out of her state of primary maternal preoccupation and becomes more attuned to her own needs and less responsive to the infant's needs, the infant begins to experience disillusionment. If the mothering takes place in an optimal fashion (what Winnicott referred to as "good enough mothering"), this process of disillusionment is always within the range of the infant's tolerance and is thus not experienced as traumatic. If, however, the degree of disillusionment is not optimal, then the infant experiences an impingement on his or her own development and adapts to the mother's needs, rather than gradually learning to develop a sense of self, which synthesizes his or her own bodily felt needs. For Winnicott, as for Ferenczi, it is likely that the reemergence of buried wishes in relationship to the therapist will be followed by disappointment. Thus the critical task for the therapist is to help the patient work through this disappointment in a constructive way. This involves coming to accept one's needs and desires as valid and legitimate, while at the same time living with the pain of recognizing that they will never be met in an absolute sense.

Heinz Kohut (1984) also placed the experience of disillusionment at the center of the change process and accorded a central role in his thinking to working through empathic failures in therapy on an ongoing basis. According to him, therapeutic change parallels the healthy developmental process in that it consists of an ongoing cycle of disappointment and repair. This results in the remobilization of an arrested developmental process through which the patient can develop a healthy and cohesive sense of self. Kohut referred to the mechanism through which this takes place as one of "transmuting internalization." For him, this involves a gradual internalization of what he referred to as the "therapist's selfobject functions." Examples of these include affective attunement, validation of subjective experience, tension regulation and soothing, organization of the experience of selfhood, and recognition of uniqueness (Bacal & Newman, 1990). Central to Kohut's thinking is the notion that the process of "optimal frustration" plays an instrumental role in promoting this process of internalization. He believed that one cannot give up one's fantasies of a perfectly available idealized other without the experience of frustration. This line of thought can be traced back to Freud's (1917) classic paper "Mourning and Melancholia," in which he first observed that people establish an identification with abandoned attachment figures as a way of dealing with object loss. Too much frustration will, however, prevent the patient from relinquishing his or her search for the idealized other.

An optimal balance between support and frustration will allow the patient to gradually develop a realistic appreciation of the therapist's "good enough" qualities and ability to find some solace in them. The disappointment that patients experience when their therapist fails plays a critical role in terms of helping them come to terms with the reality of the therapist's limitations. In the absence of working through this disappointment in an empathic fashion, however, the risk is that patients will retreat into a type of pseudomaturity that recognizes the therapist's limitations, but masks an underlying despair about the possibility of things ever being different. This results in a shutting down of one's spontaneous vitality, yearning, and hope. When the therapist is able to empathize with this disappointment, however, patients are able to experience their disappointment as meaningful and the underlying yearning and desire as valid. This is critical because it promotes a growing acceptance of their own feelings and needs. At the same time, they are able to experience the therapist as being there for them in a certain way, despite the fact that he or she is not able to fulfill their fantasies of the ideal therapist.

SUBJECTS AND OBJECTS

In a healthy development process, the individual, to some extent, comes to accept the independent existence of the other. One comes to accept the other's status as a subject rather than an object of one's needs, without having to stifle one's own creativity and bodily-felt needs in order to maintain contact with the other. While in some cases this disillusionment process of coming to terms with the separate existence of the other is less traumatic than in others, it never takes place completely smoothly. To varying degrees, then, individuals spend their lives struggling to maintain a sense of self as a vital, alive, and real subject at the same time they struggle to maintain a sense of others as real, independent subjects. To varying degrees, people continue to relate to others as objects, as characters in their own dramas, rather than as independent subjects. People try to control and possess others by trying to squeeze them into forms that fit their own fantasies and needs. In Martin Buber's (1958) terms, people relate to others as "It's" rather than as "Thou's."

The problem here is twofold. First, the world and the people in it stubbornly refuse to conform to the shapes that we try to assign to them. There is thus a constant experience of disappointment. Second, to the extent that we do treat people as objects and fail to recognize their status as subjects, we deprive them of the independent existence necessary for them to be able to provide relief from our experience of isolation and to confirm us as subjects.

Therapeutic alliance ruptures highlight the tensions that are inherent in negotiating relationships with others and bring into relief the inevitable barriers to authentic relatedness. They highlight the reality of the patient's separateness and lack of omnipotence. As we have argued, expressing one's disappointment to a therapist who accepts this criticism and survives is an important part of the process of developing a sense of agency. Learning to will or to express one's will, however, is only half the battle. The other half consists of coming to accept that the world and the people in it exist independent of one's will, that the events in the world run according to their own plan, and that other people have wills of their own. As Winnicott (1965) pointed out, an important part of the maturational process consists of seeing that the other is not destroyed by one's aggression, since this establishes the other as having a real, independent existence as a subject, rather than as an object. While this type of learning is a difficult and painful part of the disillusionment process, it ultimately helps to establish the other as capable of confirming oneself as real. In this way, the groundwork is laid for relationships in which reciprocal confirmation can take place.

The processes of coming to accept both self and other are thus mutually dependent ones that can be facilitated by working through ruptures in the therapeutic alliance. The therapist, by empathizing with the patient's experience of and reaction to the rupture, demonstrates that potentially divisive feelings (e.g., anger, disappointment) are acceptable and that experiencing nurturance and relatedness are not contingent on disowning part of oneself. He or she demonstrates that relatedness is possible in the very face of separateness and that nurturance is possible even though it can never completely fill the void that is part of the human condition. If the therapist is *good enough*, the patient will gradually come to accept her with all of her imperfections. The exploration and working through of alliance ruptures thus paradoxically entails an exploration and affirmation of both the separateness and the potential togetherness of self and other. As the patient increasingly comes to accept her own separateness and the separateness of the therapist, she has less of a desperate need to maintain some semblance of relatedness at all costs. This in turn allows her to have more authentic moments of relatedness in which she relates to the therapist in a more spontaneous way and comes closer to accepting the therapist as he is, rather than as a character in her own drama. This helps to develop an appreciation of what is referred to in the Zen tradition as "suchness," that is, an acceptance and appreciation of things as they are. This is not a passive acceptance of whatever transpires, but rather a letting go of one's attempts to manipulate self and others in pursuit of perfection. As patients' acceptance of their own fundamental aloneness, as well as their faith that moments of contact or encounter are possible, increase, they become less relentless in their pursuit of relatedness, and this permits them to be receptive to true moments of nurturance and relatedness when they do emerge. To quote Buber (1923), "The Thou meets me through grace—it is not found by seeking. But my speaking of the primary word to it as an act of my being, is indeed *the* act of my being" (p. 11).

Now let's return to the case of Benjamin. At first, he compared his therapist unfavorably to a therapist with whom he had previously consulted and who had seemed to him to be more "potent." He had experienced this other therapist as more confrontative and imagined that he had the capacity to help him achieve the type of dramatic breakthrough that did not seem forthcoming with his current therapist. At the same time, Benjamin admitted to terminating treatment with the other therapist because he felt frightened by him. Still, his disappointment in his current therapist's failure to deliver something more substantial continued to be an ongoing theme. As their relationship evolved, however, and he was able to confront the therapist with his complaints about his limitations without destroying him, he gradually came to feel more tolerant and accepting of him. As his stance toward his therapist softened, his stance toward himself softened as well, and he was gradually able to acknowledge his pain and longing for nurturance and support more directly. He spoke of feeling like a pariah because of his failure to establish a long-term relationship, and the therapist was able to feel genuinely caring for and connected to him in his despair. After one session in which his therapist had been particularly moved by his sadness, he remarked, "You know, you haven't delivered the magic I've been looking for, but somehow that feels okay right now. I don't feel so alone anymore."

NEED VERSUS NEEDINESS

An important clinical distinction can be made between "need" and "neediness" (Ghent, 1992, 1993; Shabad, 1993). When an individual has had a developmental history in which the instinctive needs for nurturance and love are responded to with neglect or punishment, she often becomes critical of her own needs and to varying degrees dissociates them. This can make it impossible for her to express her needs directly and can perpetuate a relational pattern in which her needs go unmet. In this circumstance, one often becomes resentful and indignant not only because of the initial deprivation, but also because of the ongoing failure of others to meet one's needs, and experiences a sense of entitlement, a sense that one deserves to be compensated for the deprivation one has experienced. Some of the more difficult impasses in therapy result from an enactment of such a relational pattern.

As both Ferenczi (1931) and Winnicott (1965) have suggested, the individual relates to others with a false self in order to buy time until the situation emerges where the possibility of real, authentic interpersonal contact exists. Because of the emotional deprivation the individual has experienced and because of the ongoing experience of failure to establish real contact, he seeks desperate solutions to either maintain or establish some semblance of contact and to avoid the possibility of further rejection. The very solution that the individual attempts, however, ultimately impedes real relatedness (Safran & Segal, 1990; Wachtel, 1977). The individual who, for example, because of consistent misattunement as a child, has difficulty fully experiencing and expressing sadness, will continue to experience misattunement to such feelings for others. This will create a barrier to relatedness, which may leave him or her feeling deprived and angry. Others, in turn, may be alienated by and fail to empathize with this anger. The situation can be further complicated if the individual, for fear of alienating others, expresses angry feelings in an indirect or passive–aggressive way. This can create yet another barrier that may make it difficult to establish rewarding relationships in everyday life and to establish or maintain an alliance in therapy.

This distinction between need and neediness can be further clarified with reference to Lester Luborsky's (1984) Core Conflictual Relationship Theme (CCRT) method. From Luborsky's perspective, dysfunctional relational patterns, or vicious circles, are conceptualized as consisting of three components: an underlying wish, a characteristic response of others, and a characteristic response to the self. The *wish* consists of what the individual initially wants or needs from the other—for example, the desire for comfort or nurturance. The *response of other* can be broken into two subcomponents. The first is the *expected response of other.* For example, the individual expects that others will abandon him if he expresses his need. This is based upon the individual's particular developmental experiences and is perpetuated by his or her characteristic relational matrix. The second subcomponent is the *actual response of other* and consists in this example of the act of abandonment. The *response of self* consists of the individual's response to both his expectation or internalization of the other's response and to the other's actual response. For example, the individual becomes self-critical, resentful, and indignant.

In this conceptualization, what Emmanuel Ghent (1992, 1993) refers to as "need" would be the underlying wish in Luborsky's framework. The direct expression of an underlying wish for support or nurturance has a spontaneous quality to it. Such expressions of need are experienced by others as noncoercive and tend to naturally elicit the nurturance that is sought. "Neediness," on the other hand, would be conceptualized as a response of self, a response to one's own self-criticism and expectation of abandonment. The expression of "neediness" tends to be experienced by others as demanding, coercive, and impossible to satisfy. As Ghent (1992) puts it:

What looks like need is a manipulative, at times vengeful demand-ingness, which is, in large measure, an expression of rage at lifelong de-privation of one form or another. Far from aiming to secure an appropriate response to real need, it is directed either at obtaining some immediate satisfaction, which, contributing nothing nourishing to the inner feeling of emptiness, only amplifies the feeling of depriva-tion, or at provoking the alienation or empathic remove of the other, thereby adding yet another notch in the tally of deprivations. (p. 142)

Some of the most difficult therapeutic impasses occur when thera-pists become embedded in vicious cycles of hostility and counter-hostility as they respond to patients' needy and indignant demands for help with feelings of impotence, inadequacy, and defensive outrage. What is perhaps most critical in this distinction between need and neediness is the recognition that the expression of neediness, while in-terpersonally noxious and destructive, signals the presence of an un-derlying need that is healthy and adaptive in nature. It is important to recognize that the patient's "neediness" can never be satisfied and that the process of attempting to satisfy it will only result in frustration and resentment in therapists because of the patient's failure to appreciate their efforts.

In situations of this type, what is most important is for therapists to work to understand the patient's experience empathically, and simul-taneously to strive to recognize and acknowledge when they have be-come embedded in the patient's relational matrix and are responding to neediness with frustration and anger. Although it is inevitable that therapists will at times respond aggressively and defensively, their on-going willingness to examine their contributions to the relationship and to continue to work on the patient's behalf helps the patient to be-come more trusting over time, which will eventually facilitate the emer-gence of the underlying need. In addition, it is critical for therapists to be sensitive to any incipient emergence of underlying need and to be ready to empathize and validate it when it emerges.

SURVIVING AND CONTAINING

As Winnicott (1947) suggested, there are some situations in which the most important thing the therapist can do for the patient is to survive his or her anger or destructiveness. To tolerate the patient's critical and angry feeling is a difficult task, and it is inevitable that therapists will respond as human beings with their own anger and defensiveness. The most important principle is for therapists to stay mindful and aware of the difficult feelings that are emerging in them as they experience themselves as the object of the patient's anger and to be willing to acknowledge their contributions to the interaction on an ongoing basis. The task in this context is not to avoid or to transcend angry or defensive feelings, but rather to demonstrate a consistent willingness to stick with the patient and to work toward understanding what is going on between them in the face of whatever feelings emerge for both of them.

Surviving the patient's anger does not mean never responding in anger or with hurt, nor does it mean always responding in a graceful or stylish fashion. In fact, there are times when the therapist's hurt or angry response to the patient's provocations can play an important role in helping the patient to experience the therapist as another subjectivity or to gain some sense of his or her own potency. Moreover, the process of observing the therapist struggle to deal with intense, conflicting feelings can provide a useful model for patients (Carpy, 1989; Slochower, 1997).

In a related vein, Weiss and colleagues (1986) suggest that patients who have been traumatized by the actions of others will attempt to master their traumatic feelings by acting toward the therapist as they themselves have been acted upon. They describe this as "turning passive into active." They further suggest that this constitutes a type of transference test in that the patient unconsciously hopes that the therapist will be able to deal with the painful feelings evoked in him without being traumatized, thereby providing the patient with a vicarious experience of mastering the trauma.

As discussed earlier, Bion's (1962) notion of containing can also provide a useful way of understanding the process through which surviving the patient's aggression can be therapeutic. While concepts such as turning passive into active and containing can lend themselves to defensive reification, they also point to the importance of a subtle, affective dimension of the therapeutic process when dealing with ruptures, which has nothing to do with words.

Therapists and patients are always reading and influencing one another on unconscious affective levels. What may be most critical during difficult therapeutic interactions is not the specifics of what the therapist says, but rather his or her ability to respond to the patient's unbearable feelings with his or her own sense that they are bearable and not catastrophic. In order for this to take place, therapists need to be able to experience as tolerable the feelings evoked in them by the patient's intense emotions. The processes of surviving and containing can thus be understood in terms of a form of affective communication through which the therapists help patients learn to tolerate and regulate their own affective experience. This, in turn, helps patients to harness their own affective experience in a constructive fashion and to develop the capacity to get their needs met in interpersonal relationships.

Ogden (1994) suggests that in some situations it may be preferable for the therapist to make a "silent interpretation," rather than an overt one, since any overt interpretation may be experienced as noxious by the patient in this context. It may be preferable for the therapist (at least during an initial phase) to be silent and to formulate his or her understanding to him- or herself, since any overt interpretation runs the risk of being defensively motivated if the therapist has not adequately processed his or her own feelings (e.g., Gabbard, 1996; Slochower, 1997).

As we see it, what is critical in this process is not the accuracy of the silent interpretation, but the role that it plays in helping the therapist to tolerate his or her own distressing feelings; and to the extent that a silent interpretation has a defensive element to it, it will interfere with the containment process.

There is a tendency to frame things in terms of whether it is better in a given situation for the therapist to provide a containing or a holding function, or to introduce an outside perspective in the form of interpretation or some other intervention, for example, self-disclosure (e.g., Bass, 1996; Slochower, 1996). This, however, may be an unnecessarily dichotomous way of viewing things. What is most important from our perspective is for therapists to engage in an ongoing process of self-exploration and to be vigilant for any indications of deterioration in the quality of relatedness, as they are communicating with their patients in an attempt to clarify what is being enacted. As Glen Gabbard (1996) points out, containment should not be equated with a type of passive inaction. "It involves silent processing, but it also entails verbal clarifications of what is going on inside the patient and what is transpiring in the patient–analyst dyad" (p. 198).

While it is important not to think about the issue in dichotomous terms, it is also important to recognize that during important phases of the treatment for some patients and at some points of the treatment for many patients, it becomes critical for therapists to attempt to operate predominantly from within their patients' subjective frame of reference and to manage their own conflicting feeling internally. This is particularly likely to be the case with patients whose sense of self is so fragile that the therapist's attempt to introduce his subjectivity will be experienced as a traumatic impingement (see Bach, 1985).

✳ 4

Therapeutic Metacommunication
Mindfulness in Action

In this chapter, we outline some of the key principles involved in disembedding from a relational configuration when there is a therapeutic impasse. Our focus will be on the process of metacommunication. *Metacommunication* consists of an attempt to step outside of the relational cycle that is currently being enacted by treating it as the focus of collaborative exploration: that is, communicating *about* the transaction or implicit communication that is taking place. This can be thought of as a type of *mindfulness in action*. It is an attempt to bring ongoing awareness to bear on the interactive process as it unfolds. Our thinking as presented in this chapter has been influenced by the work of a number of theorists, particularly Darlene Ehrenberg (1992), Christopher Bollas (1987), Michael Tansey and William Burke (1989), Karen Maroda (1991), and Donald Kiesler (1996), from whom we borrow the term *metacommunication* in this context. In a sense, all transference interpretations can be conceptualized as a form of metacommunication insofar as they are attempts to communicate about and make sense of what is being enacted in the therapeutic relationship. The particular form of metacommunication that we discuss here, however, has a number of distinctive features that set it apart from a more traditional transference interpretation.

Interpretations that are offered in the context of a therapeutic impasse too often are delivered in a critical and blaming fashion that reflects therapists' frustrations and their attempts to locate responsibility for the impasse in the patient, rather than in the therapeutic relationship (see Strupp, 1993). Moreover, they are particularly likely to be experienced by patients as blaming, since the therapeutic alliance is already strained. Therefore, it is especially important for any type of intervention delivered in this context to be offered in the spirit of collaborative inquiry.

In classical psychoanalytic theory, the therapist's interpretation was viewed as a communication to the patient that conveyed objective information about the patient's unconscious motivations, defenses, and relational patterns. Contemporary psychoanalytic theory is increasingly moving toward a view of things in which interpretations are understood as complex relational events, which are inevitably expressions of the therapist's subjectivity (Aron, 1996; Mitchell, 1993). Interpretations implicitly say something about the patient–therapist relationship and position the therapist vis-à-vis the patient in a particular fashion. In this respect, interpretations are speculations, conjectures, and suggestions the therapist offers to the patient in the hope of inviting him or her to engage in a collaborative process of meaning construction.

A number of contemporary theorists (e.g., Bollas, 1987) suggest that it can be helpful for therapists to share with their patients the inner process through which they arrived at a particular interpretation, in order to highlight the subjectivity of their perceptions and encourage their patients to engage in an intersubjective discourse. In a related vein, there has been a general shift away from the view that therapist's feelings are countertransference reactions that need to be privately analyzed, in order to prevent them from interfering with the therapy, toward a view in which they are valued as an important source of information. Moreover, a number of theorists now advocate disclosing countertransference feelings to the patient in order to facilitate the therapeutic process (e.g., Aron, 1996; Bollas, 1987; Ehrenberg, 1992; Maroda, 1991).

A number of contemporary analysts have even objected to the use of the term "interpretation" because it can have the connotation of an authoritative therapist conveying objective information to a less knowledgeable patient. We agree with Aron (1996) that the term does not have to be problematic as long as one keeps in mind that an interpretation is only *one individual's subjective attempt to make sense of something.* Nevertheless, we believe that the term "metacommunication" more fully captures the spirit of the type of collaborative exploration that we will focus on in this chapter.

Unlike transference interpretations, in which therapists offer conjectures about the meaning of the current interaction, metacommunication efforts attempt to decrease the degree of inference and are as much as possible grounded in the therapist's immediate experience of some aspect of the therapeutic relationship (either the therapist's own feelings or immediate perception of some aspect of the patient's actions). For example, the therapist may say, "I feel shut out by you" or "I feel like it would be easy to say something that would offend you." Countertransference disclosure plays an important role in metacommunication, but other forms of feedback are also used. For example, the therapist may say, "I experience you as withdrawn right now" or "I have an image of the two of us fencing." The objective of statements of this type is to articulate one's *implicit* or intuitive sense of something that is taking place in the therapeutic relationship in order to initiate an *explicit* exploration of that which is being unwittingly enacted.

In the next section, we provide a number of brief clinical vignettes illustrating the process of metacommunication. We then spell out the underlying principles in a systematic fashion.

CLINICAL VIGNETTES

Roxanne was a graduate student in anthropology. There was something the therapist found very likeable about her, something solid, mature, and open. She seemed to have a genuine desire to understand herself and to make use of the work with her therapist. She began therapy because of her ambivalent feelings about her husband, whom she had married 2 years earlier. Although she cared deeply about him and felt he was a wonderful husband, she believed their relationship lacked passion and she did not know whether she was ready to have children with him.

The first few months of therapy went very well. A therapeutic alliance was quickly established, and the therapist found himself looking forward to her visits. He developed a sense that they were in tune with one another; in fact, he had noted to himself, with interest, that on more than one occasion they seemed to be unconsciously swiveling their chairs back and forth in rhythm with one another, as if in reflection of their mutual attunement. As therapy proceeded, the therapist gradually realized that he was no longer looking forward to their meetings to the same extent. Although he still found himself liking Roxanne and felt that she continued to work hard in treatment, he became aware of a subtle flatness to their sessions. He was perplexed by the negative feeling, since on the face of things therapy was proceeding well, and there was nothing obvious to account for it. In an attempt to clarify what was going on, he eventually said to Roxanne: "You know, I've been trying to figure out what's going on between us. It feels to me like there's been a quality of flatness to our last few sessions. I think I've been kind of hesitant to bring it up, because of a reluctance to spoil things between us, and because I've had a sense of things going well between us, and of enjoying our time together."

In response, she was able to acknowledge her own awareness of the flatness and a similar fear of doing anything that might spoil the relationship. This metacommunication led to an exploration of the way in which she tended to present those aspects of herself to him that she believed were more admirable and likeable and had difficulty acknowledging and expressing discordant aspects of self-experience. This in turn led to an exploration of feelings of disappointment that after 6 months of treatment she was still feeling stuck in her relationship with her husband.

Larry was a 30-year-old accountant who entered treatment for long-standing depression after a brief hospitalization. He had been referred by a psychiatrist (and had refused medication). He had been in a previous psychotherapy that had ended badly around the time of his hospitalization and referral to the psychiatrist. Larry lived a very private and secluded existence. He lived alone, and had only a few acquaintances with whom he socialized on occasion. He spent most of his free time browsing the Internet and entering chat rooms. Both his parents were dead. His father passed away 10 years ago, his mother 5 years ago. He had no siblings.

What was initially striking in the treatment was the way in which Larry moved in and out of states of self-loathing (seeing himself as "pathetic") and despair. When the therapist noted these transitions and inquired about them, Larry was moved to tears and could speak no more. Typically, the first 15 minutes of their sessions were painfully awkward and uncomfortable. The therapist would ask what had happened between sessions, to which Larry responded with short, clipped remarks. When the therapist probed for Larry's experience, sometimes nothing would emerge for him and if something did emerge, he would eventually dismiss it with the comment "What's the point?" Most of the time, the probing just led to more self-consciousness, more discomfort, more paralysis, and more silence. And the more the therapist tried to metacommunicate about what was going on, the worse the situation seemed to get. The therapist soon felt that his inquiries were intrusive and just made Larry feel more pathetic and more cynical about the process. But when he chose to be silent and not force the dialogue, that just elicited frustration and more cynicism from Larry.

Increasingly, the therapist became aware of his own anxiety, his own feelings of paralysis and helplessness. He finally metacommunicated: "I'm aware of feeling paralyzed myself. I'm stuck between pursuing you, which seems to make you more anxious, and waiting for you, which seems to make you angry." This disclosure helped Larry to acknowledge that on one hand he wanted the therapist to pursue him as a demonstration of how much he cared and to admit that he felt abandoned when he didn't. On the other hand, he acknowledged experiencing the therapist's probes as a form of pressure. He was also able to acknowledge his difficulty in disclosing more of his experience on an ongoing basis because of a fundamental hopelessness about the therapist truly being there for him. This disclosure moved Larry to tears as he recalled feeling rejected and abandoned by his previous therapist. This in turn led to a deeper exploration of Larry's wish for greater intimacy and his paralyzing fear of rejection and abandonment. This mutual exploration of their shared dilemma became the first step in a shift of the relational configuration.

Susan was a depressed woman in her early 20s who was being treated concurrently with antidepressants. She had been treated successfully once before with antidepressants, but had experienced a relapse for no clearly identifiable psychological or environmental reasons. She was extremely ambivalent about being in psychotherapy, since she felt that this implied that she was to blame for her problems. On more than one occasion she asked her therapist whether he felt she should be on antidepressants; he sensed that she was testing him to see if he was willing to accept that her depression was biological and therefore beyond her control. The therapist attempted to explore the meaning of her question with her and also to convey that he would support whatever she decided, but she seemed to regard any attempt to explore her experience as intrusive and any attempt to reassure her as hollow.

During exchanges of this type, the therapist always felt cautious, unspontaneous, and concerned about saying the wrong thing. On one occasion an image came into his mind of two people playing chess, and he said to her: "It feels to me as if we're two chess players, carefully sizing one another up and trying to decide their next move. Do you know what I mean?" After she acknowledged that the image fit for her as well, he asked her what it felt like to be playing chess with him. This led to an exploration of her need to act with extreme caution in order to protect herself from him, and this in turn helped her to begin to explore her deep mistrust and feelings of vulnerability.

Emily was a 35-year-old physician who entered therapy after ending a 5-year relationship when she discovered that her boyfriend had no desire to get married and start a family. She described her relationship with her mother as strained and her relationship with her older brother as estranged. She had had a terrible fight with her brother 10 years earlier and not seen or talked to him since. Both her mother and brother abused alcohol. Her brother never completed college and had never held a steady job. Her father committed suicide when she was 10. The circumstances surrounding her father's death, as well as feelings about it, were never discussed among Emily, her mother, and her brother—there was "a conspiracy of silence," as she came to call it in therapy. After her father's death, her mother returned to work and turned to drink. Her brother proceeded to get in and out of trouble in school, but Emily, as her mother would often say about her, did "the right thing." She worked her way to a medical degree.

When she first began therapy, Emily talked much about her frustrating communications with her mother and her intolerance of "entitled" coworkers who work the system and do not do the right thing. Treatment seemed to proceed smoothly (perhaps too smoothly). Emily seemed willing and able to grapple with her perfectionism and overdeveloped work ethic and to examine her recently failed relationship and ask herself why it took 5 years to discover that her boyfriend had different aspirations. Over the first few months of treatment, she seemed moderately responsive to the therapist's interventions and reasonably satisfied with the treatment. The therapist had a sense on the edge of awareness, however, that all was not well. He was not able to articulate his concerns to himself more fully, though, and did not find himself compelled to do so.

One day, just before the start of a session, it occurred to him that Emily did not occupy much of his attention between sessions. He began to wonder to what extent he took her too lightly. He decided to explore this feeling in session, first by seeing whether he could ground it in the specifics of how they interacted and then by metacommunicating: "You know, it recently dawned on me that I rarely think or worry about you between sessions. And I became concerned that I might be taking you for granted. Does that make any sense to you?" This stirred a tearful reaction in Emily, as she acknowledged feeling neglected by the therapist. In the exploration that ensued, she associated the way in which she had always felt compelled to be self-reliant and began to identify the ways in which she tended to smooth things over and communicate that all was fine when it wasn't. She described this as a profoundly lonely experience. In time, she was able to explore the way in which her fear of being too demanding and of driving the other person away led her to disown her own desires. For

Emily, the expression of desire was too risky, invariably leading to conflict with explosive or tragic consequences.

Sam was a middle-aged writer who initially sought treatment because of writer's block and an associated depression. From the beginning, his therapist was struck with his thoughtfulness, intelligence, and psychological maturity. He was a man who had clearly struggled in a deep way with important issues in his life and had worked out a well-articulated philosophy. During their first few sessions together, the therapist found herself greatly admiring him and also doubting her own ability to help him. In an attempt to explore what might be going on in their relationship, she said to him: "You know, I find myself really admiring you. You've obviously thought about things deeply, and I find myself respecting your wisdom. At the same time, I find myself wondering if anything I could say or do would be of value to you. There is a way in which you seem to be generating your own answers as you raise the questions, and you seem very self-sufficient to me." This began to open the door to a core relational theme for him. Over time he was able to talk about his fundamental sense that others could not be counted on and that he ultimately would have to look after himself. Related to this was the link between his self-esteem and experiencing himself as wise, and the difficulty involved in seeking help from another, since this inevitably would threaten his self-esteem.

PRINCIPLES OF METACOMMUNICATION

In the rest of this chapter, we spell out the principles of metacommunication. We begin by discussing *general principles*. These are principles that outline a general orientation and view of things that provides a good foundation for metacommunication. These will be organized into three types: (1) how the therapist should participate with the patient and orient him- or herself to the alliance rupture or therapeutic impasse, (2) what the therapist should attend to and focus on, and (3) what the therapist should expect while working through a therapeutic impasse. We then outline a number of *specific principles*. These are principles that more directly spell out the steps involved in metacommunication.

General Principles

Participation and Orientation

   Principle 1. Explore with Skillful Tentativeness. Always communicate observations in a tentative and exploratory fashion (see Gendlin, 1968;

Rogers, 1951). The message at both explicit and implicit levels should always be one of inviting the patient to engage in a collaborative attempt to understand what is taking place, rather than one of conveying information with an objective status. It is critical to remember that the relational implications of a communication are as important as, if not more important than, its content (Aron, 1996; Mitchell, 1988). The tentative and exploratory nature of the therapist's intervention should be genuinely felt by the therapist, not simulated. Patients can distinguish between genuine and false humility. It is thus critical that therapists approach the situation from a stance of genuine uncertainty.

Principle 2. Establish a Sense of "We-ness." The implicit message should always be one of inviting the patient to join the therapist in an attempt to understand their shared dilemma. During periods of therapeutic impasse, patients typically feel alone and demoralized. The therapist becomes one in an endless succession of figures who are unable to join with the patient in his or her struggle. The therapist becomes another foe rather than an ally. By framing the impasse as a shared experience, the therapist begins the process of transforming the struggle by acknowledging that the therapist and the patient are stuck together.

Principle 3. Do Not Assume a Parallel with Other Relationships. The question of the extent to which an identified pattern in the therapeutic relationship generalizes to other relationships in the patient's life should always be kept an open one. It is important for therapists to communicate to patients at the outset their belief that some of the patterns taking place in the therapy are generalized to other situations, while others may not be. This stance helps them to approach patients in a nonblaming fashion and to accept responsibility for their own contribution to the interaction. Patients will thus be better able to explore their own contributions in a nondefensive fashion. The goal is to explore the particularities of the patient's internal experience and actions in a subtly nuanced fashion, as they emerge in the here-and-now, rather than to identify a more generalized relational pattern. The therapist's premature attempts at pattern identification are typically experienced as blaming by the patient. Moreover, they are often defensively motivated. When therapists explore what is going on in the here-and-now of therapeutic relationship with a genuine openness to discovering their own contributions, patients often spontaneously search for generalized patterns.

Principle 4. Emphasize One's Own Subjectivity. All metacommunication should emphasize the subjectivity of the therapist's perception (see Kiesler, 1996). This plays a critical role in establishing a climate that emphasizes the subjectivity of all perceptions and the importance of engaging in an ongoing collaborative effort to clarify what is taking place. Bollas (1987) has similarly spoken about the importance of therapists announcing their subjectivity to their patients. He suggests such simple strategies as beginning one's comments with phrases such as "What occurs to me . . . " or "I'm thinking that. . . . " Examples of other phrases that highlight the subjective nature of the therapist's interventions include "As I see it . . ., " "It seems to me . . ., " or "My sense is. . . ." Emphasizing the subjectivity of the therapist's observations also helps to establish a more egalitarian role relationship. This can be particularly important when the alliance is strained and patients are more likely to experience the therapist's intervention as controlling or assaultive. When the subjectivity of the therapist's observations is emphasized, patients are more likely to feel free either to make use of them or not and are less likely to feel a need to cling to their own perspectives and defensively reject the therapist's.

Principle 5. Emphasize Awareness Rather Than Change. When conveying feedback about behavior or an interpersonal style that is problematic or that disrupts relatedness (e.g., a contemptuous look or an intellectualized avoidance), the message that should be conveyed is one of awareness, rather than of change. Instead of conveying the message to patients that their style should change, the intent of the feedback is to bring it to their awareness and to stimulate a curiosity about the internal experience associated with their style. This emphasis is consistent with one of the fundamental principles of mindfulness—that change emerges out of nonjudgmental awareness, rather than through trying to force things to be different.

Principle 6. Ground All Formulations in Awareness of One's Own Feelings. Therapists should try to ground their formulations about the patient in awareness of their own feelings. Any formulation not grounded in this way is at increased risk for being distorted. One of the central factors in keeping therapists embedded is their inability to become aware of and acknowledge their own feelings and their unwitting participation in an enactment.

Principle 7. Start Where You Are. Metacommunication should always emerge out of the inspiration of the moment. It should be based upon feelings and intuitions that are emerging for the therapist in that moment. What was true in one session may not be true in the next one, and what was true at the beginning of a session may not be true later in that same session. Furthermore, what is true for one therapist in relationship to a particular patient will not necessarily be true for another. Thus, for example, when in supervision, it is important not to simply try to apply supervisors' or colleagues' formulations or to implement their suggestions, but rather to become more aware of one's own experience in relationship to the patient. While an observer watching a videotape of a therapy session with a hostile patient may be able to empathize with the patient's underlying vulnerability, this will be of no help to the therapist who is embedded in a particular relational configuration. Therapists must begin by accepting and working through their own feelings in the immediacy of the moment, rather than trying to be somewhere they are not.

Principle 8. Accept Responsibility for One's Own Contribution to the Interaction. Therapists should always accept responsibility for their contributions to the interaction. Bear in mind that as therapists we are always unwittingly contributing to the interaction with the patient (Aron, 1996; Jacobs, 1986; Levenson, 1972; Mitchell, 1988; Renik, 1995). The task is thus one of working in an ongoing fashion to clarify the nature of this contribution. In many cases, the process of explicitly acknowledging one's contribution to the patient can be a particularly potent intervention. First, this process can help patients to become aware of inchoate feelings that they are having difficulty articulating, in part because of fear of the interpersonal consequences. For example, acknowledging that one has been criticizing a patient can help him or her to acknowledge the resulting hurt and resentment. Second, the process of explicitly acknowledging one's contribution to the interaction can validate patients' conscious and unconscious perceptions of what is taking place and help them to trust their own judgment. Since patients often accurately perceive ways in which therapists contribute to the interaction, but have difficulty articulating their perceptions, the process of explicitly acknowledging one's contribution as a therapist can play an important role in decreasing the type of mystification that has been common in the patient's interpersonal relationships. Third, by validating the patients' perceptions through this type of acknowledgment, therapists can reduce the patients' self-doubt, thereby decreasing their need for defensiveness and paving the way for the exploration and acknowledgment of the patient's contribution to the interaction.

Attention and Focus

Principle 1. Focus on the Here-and-Now. The focus should be on the here-and-now of the therapeutic relationship and on the present moment, rather than on events that have taken place in the past (i.e., either in previous sessions or at different points in the same session). There is a tendency for both patients and therapists to deflect the focus from the here-and-now of the therapeutic relationship because it is too anxiety-provoking. Commenting on what is happening in the moment facilitates the process of mindfulness for patients. To the extent that therapists are able to comment on whatever is happening in the moment, it will become easier for patients to develop a grounded experiential awareness of both their actions and the internal experiences associated with those actions. It also helps to challenge their existing relational schemas by drawing their awareness to any therapist actions that are discrepant with their expectations.

Principle 2. Focus on the Concrete and Specific. The focus should be concrete and specific, rather than general. Whenever possible, questions, observations, and comments should focus on concrete instances. Concreteness promotes experiential awareness, rather than abstract, intellectualized speculation. Thus, for example, if in the context of exploring what is happening in the therapeutic relationship, the patient says, "I tend to back away from expressing negative feelings," the therapist can ask, "Are you aware of avoiding expressing negative feelings right now with me?" When providing therapeutic feedback, rather than saying, "You tend to speak in a very abstract way," the therapist can say, "What you're saying right now seems kind of abstract to me." When patients' attention is directed to the concrete and specific, they can make their own discoveries rather than buying into the therapist's version of reality. This type of concreteness and specificity helps them to become observers of their own behavior. It thus promotes the type of mindfulness that fosters change.

Principle 3. Gauge Intuitive Sense of Relatedness. Therapists should monitor their intuitive sense of emotional closeness with or distance from patients on an ongoing basis. This continuous assessment is one of the most important sources of diagnostic information, since it provides information about the quality of relatedness with patients in a given moment. This quality of relatedness reflects an ongoing interplay between interpersonal and intrapsychic dimensions. To the extent that patients are feeling safe, accepted and validated by the therapist, they will find it easier to access their inner experience in a genuine fashion. Conversely, to the extent that they are in contact with their inner experience, therapists will experience a greater sense of relatedness to them. A sudden shift in the direction of decreased relatedness may signal that the therapist's intervention has been hindering, rather than facilitative, and indicate the need to explore the way in which the patient has construed or experienced the intervention. Conversely, a sudden shift in the direction of increased relatedness may signal that the therapist has developed a more attuned understanding of the patient's internal experience.

Principle 4. Evaluate Patients' Responsiveness to All Interventions. Therapists should monitor the quality of patient's responsiveness to interventions on an ongoing basis. Does the patient use the therapist's intervention as a stimulus for further exploration? Does he or she respond in a minimal fashion without elaboration? Does he or she not respond? Does he or she respond in a defensive or self-justifying fashion? Does he or she agree too readily in what appears to be an attempt to be a "good" patient? It is important for the therapist to attend to subtle intuitions about the quality of the patient's responsiveness. For example, a subtle quality of compliance may be difficult to operationalize, but the therapist may sense it nevertheless. The therapist may feel at some level that the patient has an ambivalent response to his or her intervention, even though he or she has difficulty articulating the relevant cues.

Principle 5. Explore Patients' Experience of Interventions. If an intervention fails to deepen exploration or further inhibits it, or if the therapist senses something peculiar in the patient's response to it, it is critical to explore the way in which the patient experienced it. Did he or she experience the therapist's intervention as critical, blaming, or accusatory? Did he or she experience it as domineering, demanding, or manipulative? Over time, this type of exploration can help to articulate the nature of the enactment taking place. It can help to articulate patients' characteristic way of construing interpersonal relationships and gradually lead to a fleshing out of their relational schemas. It can also lead to a progressive refinement in therapists' understanding of their own contribution to the interaction.

Expectation

Principle 1. Recognize That the Situation is Constantly in Flux. Bear in mind that the situation is constantly changing. What was true about the therapeutic relationship a moment ago is not true now. Therapists should try to use whatever is emerging in the present as a point of departure for further metacommunication. All situations are workable provided that one fully acknowledges and accepts what the situation is. Even the position of "being stuck" is a position that is workable once one accepts it and ceases to fight against it.

Therapists who are caught in an internal struggle in an attempt to deny their experience are too preoccupied to see ongoing changes in process. By fully acknowledging and accepting a situation, therapists can become sufficiently freed up emotionally to observe and make use of new possibilities that are emerging in the moment. The act of disclosing an experience, against which one has been fighting, can sometimes be part of the process of acknowledging and accepting one's experience (or what Neville Symington, 1983, has referred to as an "act of freedom"). For example, the therapist who says to her patient, "I feel stuck," may in the process free herself up sufficiently to see something that has eluded her before (e.g., some aspect of the patient's behavior that has been contributing to the "stuckness"). Moreover, a disclosure of this type may contribute to a shift in the interactional dynamic. For example, by acknowledging her vulnerability, the therapist may be disengaging from a power struggle, thereby making it easier for the patient to disengage. Whether or not the therapist chooses to disclose his or her current experience to a patient is not as critical as this inner act of acceptance. This inner act facilitates a type of "letting go" and an increased attunement to the unique configuration of the moment.

Principle 2. Expect Resolution Attempts to Lead to More Ruptures. No matter how hard therapists work to follow these principles, there is always a risk that any form of therapeutic metacommunication will further aggravate the alliance rupture. Metacommunication may be unconsciously motivated by anger or an attempt at self-vindication. Moreover, even in a situation in which the therapist is not metacommunicating defensively there is always a risk that it will place a greater strain on the alliance. Regardless of how skillful the therapist may be in framing his or her comments in a nonblaming, nonjudgmental way, metacommunication may be implicitly suggesting that patients should be saying or doing something other than what they are currently saying or doing. For example, the observation "I experience you as withdrawing right now" may carry with it the implication that it would be better not to withdraw.

Therapists are often reluctant to metacommunicate because of their concerns about further jeopardizing the alliance or because they feel uncomfortable with their own feelings in difficult sessions. It is important, however, to see metacommunication as one step in the process of disembedding rather than as the ultimate intervention, which is delivered once the therapist has a formulation. Viewing metacommunication this way gives therapists the freedom to be creative and experimental in their interventions. It can help to free them up when they are feeling paralyzed by their inability to understand the situation or by the perceived unacceptability of their own feelings.

Often initial attempts at metacommunication are a further manifestation of the enactment that is already taking place. For example, a
therapist, who begins to become aware of a subtle but pervasive quality
of distance in the way his patient relates to him, says: "It feels to me like
you have a subtle wall up. Do you have any sense of this?" The patient
responds to this comment by further withdrawing. It is important in
this situation for the therapist to let go of his attachment to seeing the
metacommunication work and to maintain an ongoing state of mindfulness, which will eventually allow him to develop a fuller grasp of
what is happening in the interaction.

For example, the therapist comments on the patient's continued
withdrawal as follows: "My sense is that something I said led you to
withdraw even further." He notes to himself that the patient continues
to be withdrawn. He is about to comment once again on this withdrawal, when he becomes aware of a feeling of urgency on his part.
This awareness allows him to take a step back from the interaction, and
now he begins to develop a greater sense of his contribution. He then
says: "You know, I'm beginning to get a sense that I'm battering away at
you, as if I'm trying to break down a wall." In response, the patient begins to relax and decrease his defensiveness.

The prerequisite for this last intervention is a shift in the therapist's inner state. While it can be useful to think about ways of formu-
lating interventions in a nonaccusatory way (e.g., Wachtel, 1993), it is
important to remember the ubiquitousness of the process of unconscious affective communication. The feeling behind the therapist's
words inevitably mediates their impact on the patient. In this example,
the therapist's growing awareness of his own contribution has shifted
the feeling behind his words, so that they are now no longer a manifestation of frustration, but instead a reflection of his growing empathy
for the patient's dilemma. As exemplified in this illustration, therapists' initial attempts at metacommunication can function, in part, as
an intensification of an enactment that has been taking place. When
therapists maintain an ongoing discipline of mindfulness, this intensification can make it easier for them to begin to see their own roles as
perpetrators.

Principle 3. Expect to Revisit the Same Impasse Repeatedly. It is common for the same impasse to be revisited again and again. To the extent that therapists relate to an impasse as simply a recurrence of a previous impasse, it will be impossible to relate to it in its *own* terms. It will
thus be difficult to find a way through the impasse that is grounded in
a full acceptance and appreciation of the unique configuration of the
moment. Our preconceptions can block us from mining the moment

for all its possibilities. It is thus important for therapists to attempt to approach each manifestation of an impasse with a *beginner's mind*.

Principle 4. Expect to Lose Hope. During periods of prolonged impasse, therapists can easily lose hope in the possibility of moving forward. There is no easy way to sustain hope at such times. It is important to know that periods of hopelessness and demoralization are part of the process, just as the process of working through impasses is *the* work of therapy, rather than a prerequisite. The absence of hope, paradoxically, can create a type of fertile void in which new possibilities can emerge. In the Zen tradition, it is said that enlightenment comes when one gives up all hope of things being different. T. S. Eliot (1963) captures this intuition beautifully in a passage from his poem "East Coker":

> I said my soul, be still, and wait without hope.
> For hope would be hope for the wrong thing; wait without love.
> For love would be love of the wrong thing; there is yet faith.
> But faith and the love and the hope are all in the waiting.
> Wait without thought, for you are not ready for thought:
> So the darkness shall be the light, and the stillness the dancing.
> (pp. 126–127)

Specific Principles

In this section, we outline a number of specific principles of metacommunication under the separate headings of *awareness* and *communication*. In some respects, the process of becoming aware of one's experience as the therapist precedes the process of communicating that awareness to the patient. At the same time, however, it is important to recognize that in practice these processes often take place simultaneously and that the act of musing out loud to the patient about the interaction often helps therapists put into words for themselves subtle perceptions that might otherwise remain at an implicit level.

Awareness

Principle 1. Awareness of Feelings, Images, and Fantasies. The first step involves identifying feelings and responses that the patient evokes in the therapist. While the identification of feelings is one of the better starting points, the identification of other internal experiences (e.g., seemingly unrelated thoughts, fantasies, or memories) can also be useful (see Ogden, 1994; Jacobs, 1991). One should bear in mind that this identification requires a careful exploration of the nuances of therapists' experience, and that it may take some time before they can begin to articulate their own experience to themselves. While in some situations therapists may want to partially articulate their experience to themselves before they make any interventions based on them, in other situations the process of articulating this experience to the patient is an important part of the process of clarifying it for themselves.

Principle 2. Awareness of Action Tendencies. In many situations, it is easier for therapists to identify the actions they feel like taking than what they feel. For example, does the therapist feel like dominating the patient? Justifying himself? Agreeing with the patient? Trying to obtain the patient's approval? Finding fault with the patient or "puncturing his balloon?"

Principle 3. Retrospective Awareness of One's Own Actions. It is often difficult for therapists to identify the impact that the patient has on them until they have already acted. As Owen Renik (1995) has pointed out, awareness often follows action. For example, the therapist may become aware that he has been attempting to justify himself in response to the patient's criticisms. He may become aware of a critical tone in his voice when he speaks to the patient. He may become aware in retrospect that he has been acting flirtatiously toward the patient, or acting in a constrained and nonspontaneous fashion.

Principle 4. Identification of Interpersonal Markers. Therapists should try to identify specific patient behaviors and communications that may evoke or contribute to their feelings. This involves identifying the characteristic patient mannerisms that may be problematic for them in other situations. For example, a therapist feels patronized and begins to link these feelings to a condescending sound in the patient's voice and to an arrogant tilt of the head that is characteristic for him. Or the therapist continuously finds her attention wandering to other events of the day while a particular patient is talking. She begins to link these feelings to the patient's characteristic manner of speech, which tends to be general and vague.

As previously indicated, these characteristic patient mannerisms can be thought of as *interpersonal markers*. These markers are significant for a number of reasons. First, identifying them helps therapists to disembed from the relational configuration by beginning to clarify what they are reacting to. Moreover, once interpersonal markers have been identified, therapists can anticipate them rather than acting automatically. For example, a therapist who has a tremendous amount of difficulty staying awake with a particular patient begins to search for interpersonal markers that may play a role in evoking such a state. The process of actively searching, in itself, begins to shift his experience and decrease his sleepiness. He then identifies a particular tone of voice to which he may be in part responding—a type of dreamy quality that seems to say "Everything is wonderful" and at the same time conveys a sense of unreality. Identifying this marker helps him to further dis-embed.

Second, the process of identifying tangible patient behaviors and communications that may be evoking therapists' feelings helps them to further articulate their feelings. For example, in the above illustration, identifying his patient's dreamy tone of voice helps the therapist to begin to identify a feeling of irritation. It is as if his patient is denying that anything of substance goes on in her inner world when he and she both know that this is not true.

Third, interpersonal markers are potential windows into understanding patients' relational matrices (including relational schemas, characteristic patterns of relating, and characteristic responses of others). In the same way that an interpersonal marker elicits a distinctive response from the therapist, it may elicit similar responses from others. Moreover, interpersonal markers are often associated with fundamental beliefs about self and others that play an important role in shaping patients' relational matrices. They are thus an important interface between patients' internal and interpersonal worlds. For example, in the above illustration, further exploration revealed that the patient's dreamy voice was associated with an attempt to modulate painful feelings because of a fundamental belief that others (including the therapist) would not be able to tolerate them. Interpersonal markers thus provide important junctures for exploring patients' experience.

Communication

Principle 1. Disclose Experience or Acknowledge One's Own Actions. Therapists can begin the process of working through an impasse by sharing their own experience (feelings, images, fantasies, or descriptions of their own actions) with their patients. During this process, it is important to make two things clear: (1) that their experience is not simply caused by the patient, and (2) that there is no guarantee that this experience will help shed light on what is going on in the current interaction. For example, the therapist might say: "I'm aware that I've been feeling really constrained the last few minutes. I'm not sure what this may have to do with us, but if you're open to it, I'd like to explore whether this feeling has any relevance to what's going on between us."

As we previously indicated, the process of articulating one's feelings to patients can begin to free oneself to intervene more effectively. Therapists' feelings of being stuck or paralyzed often reflect difficulty in acknowledging and articulating to themselves what they are currently experiencing. Once therapists have disclosed their feelings, it is useful to follow up with a probe to explore aspects of the patient's experience that may be related to the impact that he may be having on the therapist. For example, a therapist becomes aware of feeling very cautious in his approach toward the patient and says: "I'm aware of feeling cautious in what I say to you, as if I could easily say or do the wrong thing. Does that feedback make any sense to you?"

Further, the process of acknowledging one's contributions to the patient can play a critical role in beginning to clarify the nature of the cycle that is being enacted. For example, a therapist says: "As I listen to myself talk, I hear a kind of stilted quality to what I'm saying, and I think I've probably been acting in a pretty formal and distant fashion with you. Does that fit with your experience?" If the patient is receptive, this type of disclosure can lead in the direction of either clarifying factors influencing the therapist's actions (e.g., an intuitive sense that the patient is very judgmental) or exploring the patient's feelings about the therapist's actions (e.g., an experience of disappointment or abandonment). The following vignette illustrates this process.

> Frank was a 40-year-old, married, freelance copywriter who felt frustrated with his inability to find a full-time position. He described a marriage in which his wife was frequently and intensely critical and he was avoidant and passive–aggressive. He had a 5-year-old son whom he loved dearly and who (according to Frank) kept him in the marriage. When he entered therapy, he reported struggling with bouts of anxiety and depression and with "problems in contacting, relating, and responding to others," which have debilitated him in his marriage and in his work.
>
> In therapy, Frank frequently demonstrated an avoidant, equivocating, and convoluted style of communicating. In one session, Frank became very self-critical as the therapist was pushing him to explore his anger toward his critical wife. When the therapist noted the shift in self-states and tried to draw the patient's attention to it, Frank responded in a cryptic way, making associations to feelings and memories that confused the therapist and left him at a loss as to what Frank meant. What ensued was a dogged pursuit of understanding and a torturous game of cat and mouse. The more the therapist inquired into the meaning of Frank's responses, the more convoluted they became. At some point the therapist metacommunicated his confusion. This only served to elicit greater convolution. Finally, the therapist became more aware of his own frustration and anger, of his aggression in the

interaction, and commented: "I have a sense of us playing cat and mouse where I'm aggressively pursuing and pressuring you. It just occurred to me how aggressively I'm chasing you. Is that consistent with your experience?"

In response, Frank was able to begin acknowledging his perception of the therapist's aggression. At first, this acknowledgment was very tentative, but over time Frank was able to express his anger at the therapist more directly and begin to experience the way in which his fear of retaliation contributed to a self-defeating relational matrix.

Principle 2. Link One's Own Feelings to an Interpersonal Marker. In this form of metacommunication, therapists attempt to spell out possible relationships between their own feelings and patients' interpersonal markers. This can help patients begin to develop some awareness of the way in which aspects of their characterological styles and unconscious ways of being may impact on others. For example, the therapist may say: "I'm feeling kind of shut out, and I think it has to do with the way in which you seem to dismiss whatever I say out of hand, without apparently giving it any consideration." Or she might remark: "Just now I was trying to empathize with your experience, and I felt brushed away. Did you have any awareness of doing that?" The therapist might also say: "I'm feeling kind of tongue-tied, almost reluctant to say anything, and I'm trying to figure out what's going on. I think it may be related to a look I see on your face. Just now, for example, I see a faint smile on your face that looks almost like a smirk to me. I find myself interpreting it as a look of scorn or derision. Do you have any awareness of the smirk I'm talking about?" At this point, if the patient reports having some awareness of his facial expression, the therapist can proceed to explore the experience associated with it. For example, she might say: "Any sense of what's going on for you when . . . ?" or "Any sense of the feelings connected with the smirk?" If the patient does not report an awareness of the identified interpersonal marker, it is important for the therapist to back off. She may, however, indicate that she will try to point it out the next time it comes up, in order to help the patient become aware of it. In this fashion, therapists can gradually direct the patient's attention to the identified interpersonal marker, and by repeatedly noting it when it occurs, help him or her to become aware of the dissociated experience that may be linked to it.

Principle 3. Identify an Interpersonal Marker and Explore the Experience That Is Linked to It. In this type of exploration, the therapist directly brings an identified interpersonal marker to the patient's attention without linking it to a personal feeling or reaction. This can be useful when the therapist notes a distinctive interpersonal marker that does not immediately appear to be linked to his or her own feelings or experience. For example, the therapist might remark: "I'm aware of you turning away from me as you talk about your feelings. Do you have any awareness of this?" Or the therapist might note: "I'm aware of you clenching your jaw as you talk. Do you have any awareness of this? Any sense of what your experience is as you do this?" Or the therapist might say: "I'm aware of you lowering your voice and rushing through it as you talk about this. What's happening inside?" By drawing the patient's awareness to a nonverbal behavior he or she may not be aware of, the therapist may facilitate awareness of a related experience that is dissociated. For example, the patient whose attention is directed to his clenched fist may become aware of corresponding anger, or the patient whose attention is directed to the way in which she is lowering her voice may become aware of corresponding feelings of shame.

Principle 4. Provide Feedback Regarding Subjective Experience or Perception of Patient. In this type of feedback, the therapist conveys his or her impression or intuitive sense of some aspect of the patient's current state or actions. This type of feedback is typically based on some combination of observation of the patient's nonverbal behavior and feelings that are evoked in the therapist. While in some instances therapists may wish to articulate to themselves or the patient what the impression is based on, in other cases it is sufficient to convey an intuitive impression. For example, the therapist might say: "I experience you as withdrawing right now." Or he might remark: "It feels to me like you just put up a wall." Or she might note: "It feels to me as if you're judging me right now." Or the therapist might declare: "It feels to me that you are attacking and at the same time softening the blow." As always, the therapist's tone should be tentative and exploratory in nature.

The objective of this type of feedback is to help patients become aware of an aspect of their experience or actions that they may not be fully aware of. Thus, for example, a patient who dissociates her own critical feelings may be able to use this type of feedback to begin to explore the internal experience that corresponds to the actions and subtle nonverbal communications that the therapist may be picking up on. Feedback of this type is typically followed with an exploratory probe, for example, "Does that feedback make any sense to you?" or "Does that feedback correspond to any experience that is going on inside of you?" or "Do you have any awareness of putting up a wall?" If the patient acknowledges some awareness of the experience that is being explored, the therapist can explore the experience further by asking questions such as, "What does it feel like to be putting up a wall right now?" or "What does it feel like to be skeptical right now?" Alternatively, the therapist can ask the patient to put the experience into words, for example, "Can you put your skepticism into words?"

Principle 5. Comment on What May Be a Shared Experience. In this form of feedback, the therapist comments on what may be a shared experience as a lead into exploring any patient feelings, perceptions, or attitudes that may be associated with the interaction. For example, the therapist might say: "It feels to me as if the two of us are playing chess." Or "It feels to me like the two of us are being very cautious with one another right now." Or "I have a sense that both of us are being very polite right now." Or "It feels to me like we're both being very tentative right now." Or "It feels to me like I'm constantly intruding, and you're trying to politely keep me out." If the observation resonates with the patient's experience, the therapist can ask him or her to further elaborate on the therapist's experience of the interaction. Conversely, if it fails to resonate, the therapist can ask the patient to try to put into words his or her own experience of the interaction.

Principle 6. Track the Patient's Response to an Intervention. The therapist should carefully monitor the patient's response to all interventions. It is vital to be particularly vigilant for indications that the patient experiences an intervention as critical or blaming. If the therapist feels there is any indication that his or her comment has not been facilitative, he or she should explore the way in which it was experienced by the patient. For example, the therapist might ask: "How did it feel when I said that to you?" or "I'm not sure I know what's going on for you right now. I wonder how you felt when I said that?"

Bear in mind that patients may have difficulty acknowledging feeling hurt or criticized by the therapist or feeling angry at the therapist. To do so may be threatening to their self-esteem (e.g., they believe it means they are weak) or may in their minds risk offending or alienating the therapist. When the therapist suspects that a patient has experienced the metacommunication as critical, despite the fact that he or she denies it, sometimes it can be facilitative to be more interpretive. For example, the therapist might say: "I wonder if you felt criticized or hurt by what I said."

Also, bear in mind that the patient's perception that the therapist has been critical, invalidating, or patronizing may be accurate to varying degrees. It is not uncommon for a therapist's attempt to metacommunicate or interpret to be in part fueled by negative feelings such as anger or frustration. This is particularly likely to be true when therapists are metacommunicating in an attempt to work their way out of an impasse. If the therapist becomes aware of having been critical or blaming while metacommunicating, it can be particularly useful to acknowledge it, even if the patient is not consciously aware of it or has not brought it up. For example, the therapist might say: "I have a sense that I may have sounded angry or critical when I said that. Did it sound that way to you?" or "As I listen to my voice, it sounds angry [or frustrated or critical] to me. Does it sound that way to you?" Explicitly acknowledging one's own contribution to the interaction can help patients to become more aware of their own experience. When the therapist lets go of his or her attempt to locate responsibility for the interaction in the patient, the patient in turn has less of a need to protect him- or herself through defensive maneuvers and can begin to feel safe enough to explore.

The process of exploring the patient's construal of an intervention that he or she has not experienced as facilitative can play a critical role in refining therapists' understanding of the enactment that is taking place and deepening their understanding of the patient's relational matrix. This is true for two reasons. First, clarifying the patient's construal of the intervention may help therapists to further understand their own contributions to the enactment. For example, the patient who experiences an intervention as critical may be accurately perceiving dissociated anger and frustration in the therapist. Second, exploring the patient's construal of a failed intervention may help therapists to further clarify their own understanding of the patient's relational schemas. For example, the patient may experience the therapist's intervention as an attempt to "con him," and this may related to a more generalized fear of being taken advantage of and to an underlying fear of depending on other people because of an anticipation of being disappointed and humiliated. In situations of this type, it is critical to work toward understanding the subtle nuances of the patient's idiosyncratic experience of the failed intervention, rather than to assimilate his or her experience into a preconceived understanding of what is taking place.

Principle 7. Invite the Patient to Explore the Therapist's Contribution. Another valuable intervention involves inviting patients to explore the therapist's contribution. This can consist of either inviting them to make suggestions about how the therapist's actions are contributing to the impasse or to speculate about what may be going on for the therapist internally (Aron, 1996). For example, the therapist might ask: "What is it that you see me doing that gives you that impression." Or "I wonder if you have any thoughts about what may be going on for me right now?" Or "Any thoughts about what I might be thinking or feeling?" Questions of this type help to clarify patients' construal of the therapist. This can lead to a further articulation of their relational schemas. They can also provide new insight into the therapist's own contribution to the impasse. In this regard, it is critical for therapists to be open to accepting their patient's perception and to genuinely consider its truth claim.

CLINICAL ILLUSTRATION

The following transcript illustrates the process of therapeutic metacommunication.

> The patient, Joan, was a 49-year-old woman who sought therapy because of social isolation and occupational problems resulting from severe impairments in her interpersonal functioning.

JOAN (J): So I would say that last week was sort of off track, wouldn't you?

THERAPIST (T): In what way?

J: Well, we started off by saying here's point A and here's point B, now let's get from A to B. That was fine, and everything was great, and then, of course, it all went backward again.

T: In what way did it go backward?

J: I don't know. . . . I just don't see the relevance of what we're doing.

T: Do you have a sense of what would be relevant?

J: Well . . . my occupational therapist, Sarah . . . is supposed to be working on my social skills, and you're supposed to be working on the thinking part . . . kind of a philosophy lesson. That's what I came here for.

T: Can you say any more about what that "philosophy lesson" would look like?

J: I don't know. You're the professional.

T: So you're kind of saying . . .

J: The ball's in your court, that's right, buster. I've led you by the nose as much as I can . . . I mean, cripes, you've got to do something.

T: Uh-huh.

J: If I can sit here and do it by myself, what the hell do I need you for?

T: My sense is that when I try to run with the ball, I go off course.

J: Well, you start going really . . . all over the place. I mean, you don't—you don't go deep enough. When you do pick up something . . . you don't go deep enough . . . you don't stick to it so that it gets somewhere. I mean, I know the surface stuff, and I mean, you've got to go beyond that.

T: You weren't happy with the way things went last week?

J: Well, what did I get out of it?

T: Umm . . .

J: I mean, what was there that wasn't there before?

T: You're phrasing that as a question, but I think you're also saying that you didn't get anything out of it.

J: I don't know about that. I've had the experience with Sarah of her pointing out that I'm making more progress than I think I am and then decide, "Well, maybe she's right." So if you see something that I don't, I want you to let me know.

T: So, you're inviting me to try and show you that something worthwhile did happen last week?

J: Well, you said I wasn't really asking a question before. Well . . . I want to give you an opportunity to show me I'm wrong.

T: What are the chances that I could say something that would get you to change your mind about last week?

J: Well . . . not all that high . . . but maybe you saw something I didn't.

T: See . . . my feeling is that it's tempting to try to convince you, but I have a sense that I wouldn't have much of a shot at it . . . that it would become a struggle about who's right . . . you or me?

The session begins with evidence of a clear strain in the alliance. Joan complains that their work together has gotten "off track" although she appears to have some difficulty articulating precisely how. Her statement that she wants a "philosophy lesson" suggests that she wants something more concrete, didactic, or directive from the therapist. She also appears to have the therapist assigned to a specific slot from which he is not supposed to stray. This might have been a useful focus for metacommunication (e.g., "My sense is that you assign me to a very specific slot that I'm not supposed to stray from."). But the therapist moves on and continues to attempt to clarify Joan's understanding of the tasks of therapy, since this may lead to a deeper understanding of the underlying relational theme that is being enacted. Joan's angry response (e.g., "I've led you by the nose as much as I can . . . I mean cripes . . . you've got to do something.") suggests that she experiences him as continuing to shirk his re-

sponsibilities. At this point, the therapist metacommunicates his dilemma ("My sense is that when I try to run with the ball, I go off course."). This admission leads into an interaction in which Joan attempts to get the therapist to convince her that the previous session was not wasted. Rather than responding to the pull to do so, he metacommunicates his dilemma once again ("My feeling is that it's tempting to try to convince you, but I have a sense that I wouldn't have much of a shot at it . . . that it would become a struggle about who's right . . . you or me?"). Perhaps a fuller articulation of the dilemma would be something like "I feel torn. On the one hand, I have a sense that I'm letting you down by not being more forceful. But on the other hand, I'm concerned that if I respond to the temptation to do so, we'll just get into a struggle about who's wrong and who's right."

J: Well . . . unless I missed something. Although I realize when you mention the "right" part . . . I mean . . . that's come up a couple of times before. I know I have a thing about always having to be right. But we're getting off track again. I don't think this is getting us anywhere.

T: I'm willing to follow your lead right now. What direction would you like to go in?

J: Well . . . there is something about me only being able to see things in black-and-white terms. Like I've said before, I know that's a problem for me. And I need you to help me see shades of grey.

T: Any sense of what would be a useful way of going about that?

J: Well . . . you once asked me what would happen if I were wrong, or whatever. You pursued that a little bit . . . but then you just dropped it.

T: Okay, so what would happen if you were wrong?

J: (*Pause.*) Well . . . I'd have trouble living with myself. I don't normally think of appearances being that big a deal to me, but obviously somewhere along the line I got this idea that I have to be right, and things have to be my way, or things have to be the way I think is right, which is the same, I suppose, as "my way." I mean, people say that I just need things to be my way. But I don't think that's necessarily true. I think it's more tied up with the "right and wrong" deal. Of course, I know I have trouble accepting some things I don't like, and I know what a terrific rationalizer I am . . . so I can't always be sure . . . cause I do such a good job of rationalizing that I'm not always sure what's behind the rationalizing. I believe my rationalizing. That's my defense mechanism.

T: Uh-huh. I have an impression that I think is related to the theme of "right or wrong." Are you open to some feedback?

J: Okay.

T: Okay. I get kind of a sense when you talk, right now, that it's kind of like you've got it all figured out.

J: Well . . . so I just want you to give me a new way of looking at things, so I can throw the old way out. But the new way has to be as good as the old way.

T: My feeling is that . . .

J: You don't think it's possible.

T: Well, it feels like there's no room for me to, um, really, enter into a real dialogue with you because I have a sense from you that you've got it all figured out. That you've got yourself all figured out.

J: Well, I haven't got it all figured out, because I don't know where the original way of looking at things came from.

T: Uh-huh. But what about my experience of feeling that there's no room for a dialogue?

J: I see, I see, yeah, I would say that would be a reasonable observation.

T: Uh-huh.

J: And, of course, I don't like that because then that's the same garbage that I'm getting from everybody. "Well, you don't want to change, you've already decided this," and all the rest of it. You've said it slightly different, so it's not so . . . you know . . . it's not negative the way the rest of them say it . . . so I automatically attack them and defend myself. I mean . . . you've said it so that I don't automatically attack.

T: But it still feels not so nice, huh?

J: Well, it's not nice . . . but as I said . . . it certainly sounds like a reasonable observation.

The therapist's metacommunication regarding his concerns about getting into a struggle helps to open up an exploration of Joan's need to be right all the time. At first Joan balks at the prospect of exploring this issue further by questioning the relevance of this therapeutic task. The therapist defers to her. This would be an example of indirectly addressing a strain in the alliance by agreeing to change the therapeutic task (Chapter 1). Joan responds well to this tactic

and continues to explore her need to be right all the time, although in intellec-
tualized terms. At this point, the therapist directs her attention to the way in
which her current intellectualized exploration is a manifestation of the very
theme she is talking about. His intervention has a number of important fea-
tures that are characteristic of good metacommunication. It focuses on the con-
crete and the here-and-now, it emphasizes the subjectivity of the therapist's per-
ception, and it articulates his personal experience ("Well, it feels like there's no
room for me to, um, really, enter into a real dialogue with you"). It appears
that Joan feels that she is being criticized, and he is careful to explore whether
this is the case. It seems, however, that even if she is feeling mildly criticized,
she is still able to use the therapist's comments to facilitate further exploration.

T: Well, then let me ask you a related question. Um, what would it mean to you if you didn't have it all figured out . . . if you didn't have yourself all figured out?

J: I assume I'd be in chaos. I don't know. I don't know, cause I've always been controlled. As I said, there's no room for any emotions and feelings and stuff. Everything's all cut and dried and has been ever since I can remember.

T: Okay, let me ask you . . . is this . . . do you have a sense of this as "on track" (what we're talking about now) or "off track?"

J: No, it's reasonable. I don't know if it's gonna get anywhere, but at least it's reasonable.

T: Uh-huh.

J: If you don't ask me how I feel or some other dumb, useless question. (*Pause.*) No, I think that's a very valid observation. And it does sort of make you wonder, doesn't it?

T: What does it make you wonder?

J: Well, like you said, "Where is the room for me?" You know . . . I think that's a very valid point. I think you've probably put your finger on what other people have been saying . . . but, of course, they don't say it that way . . . so therefore they probably don't even realize that's what they mean, cause they don't see it that way. But I guess I'm waiting for some magic answer that'll make me drop that and then go pick up something else. I mean, that's basically what I'm after now. Isn't it?

T: What you're saying right now sounds important to me. It's not easy for you to let go of the way you look at things . . .

J: Yeah . . . everybody gets pissed off at me and says, "We can't help you until you let go and throw away the other stuff," and my answer to that is "Well, that's exactly what happened with Fred Demos and his philosophy of religion course . . . "

T: Wait . . . wait, who's Fred Demos?

J: He's a philosophy of religion professor they had where I went to college, who was very controversial. He wanted to turn me into an agnostic, and he did that to a lot of people because he . . . he was a very good philosopher. And, and of course, a lot of the chaplains and ministers in the area had a real problem with him. My mother's comment was, "Well, that's fine, he tore it down, but he put nothing in its place, and all he did was end up leaving you with a void." And that's true. It's easy to tear stuff down . . .

T: So he took away your beliefs and left you with nothing in its place?

J: Well . . . not much. And whatever I've got left, I'm not going to let people take away from me without putting something in its place.

Joan's exploration of her need to stay in control by having all the answers begins to take on a more vulnerable, experientially grounded quality. Sensing the tenuous nature of the alliance, the therapist continues to explicitly make sure that Joan is on board with respect to the specific therapeutic task of the moment. Joan's associations lead to a painful memory of what sounds like an existential crisis during her college years. Her story of having her belief system "torn down" by her philosophy professor constitutes what Joseph Lichtenberg, Frank Lachmann, and James Fosshage (1992) refer to as a "model scene," that is, a memory that telescopes or condenses affectively and thematically similar events in the patient's life and sheds light on a core relational theme, and possibly the patient–therapist interactive matrix (see Muran, Samstag, Segal, & Winston, 1998; Tomkins, 1987). It also helps to shed some light on the meaning of Joan's earlier request for a "philosophy lesson" from the therapist.

T: Uh-huh. Does it feel like I'm trying to take something away from you?

J: Well . . . the whole profession in general.

T: Yeah?

J: People say, "If you want to change, you've got to do this, and you've got to do that. You've got to tear stuff down and throw it away." They're not saying anything positive. They're not giving me anything to work with. They're not giving me a philosophy of life as an alternative. They're giving me nothing that fits and works as well as what I've got. They say, "Well, it doesn't work, so what have you got to lose by throwing it away?" That's as stupid a thing as I've heard.

T: You know, when you speak about other people right now, rather than what's going on between you and me, it makes it difficult for me to kind of engage with you and get close to you.

J: Okay . . . well . . . you haven't tried . . . you haven't tried to do anything. I mean you're not part of the . . . you know . . . as I say . . . you and Sarah are the closest . . . you and Sarah are the only two that have understood anything, and, ah, you've never said that you thought I wasn't trying. And you don't say things just to pat me on the head and make me feel better. And you've given me reasons to back yourself up, so I could believe you. Cause I don't believe anything anybody says just for the sake of it . . . just cause they're saying it. They have to show me proof they mean what they say. I can always rationalize why people say things, but if they back it up, that shows that they mean it, and then I'll listen to it. . . . And you haven't just said things to pat me on the back . . . cause you know I don't want to hear that . . . so you haven't said it. You've backed it up with reasons why you thought that . . . so therefore I believe you.

T: Uh-huh.

J: I don't take well to people patting me on the head to try to soothe me . . . to make you look good or make me feel better.

T: Uh-huh.

J: I won't put up with that.

T: What's happening for you?

J: Nothing. . . . It's just the way I am . . . I gotta be different, I won't put up with that. Other people will . . . but I won't.

T: Let me tell you something else which is going on for me that I think is related to the same theme. What I'm doing really is looking for ways to try and get a little bit closer to you . . . sort of looking for openings that you'll allow, so I can sort of begin to really talk with you . . . you know . . . get a sense of what's really going on inside you. And every now and then my sense is that you sort of allow me in a little bit.

J: So you've got to take the chance when I give it to you.

T: Are you aware of when you allow me in a little bit and when you don't?

J: Yeah, I give people a chance. And if they're interested and if they're on the ball, they'll take it. And if they're not interested and not on the ball, they won't take it . . . so that's fine. Just brush them off and put them on the outside again.

The therapist attempts to explore the connection between Joan's feelings about her encounter with her philosophy of religion professor and the therapeutic relationship, but keeps a more generalized focus. The therapist metacommunicates his experience of feeling distanced by this. Joan appears to have difficulty directly acknowledging concerns about the therapist undermining her beliefs. Her response is a rather complex one, presumably reflecting intense conflicting emotions and her attempts to manage them. At first, it sounds like she is continuing to criticize him for not providing something more substantial ("you haven't tried to do anything"). She then transitions into expressing her appreciation of the therapist for not accusing her of resisting and for not patronizing her. Her own associations now appear to evoke feelings of anger and prideful indignation at the thought of people patronizing her. Although we can only speculate about precisely what is going on internally for Joan, at an interpersonal level it is clear that she has pulled away from the therapist again. He metacommunicates in a general way about what he is trying to do (i.e., he is looking for openings and ways of getting closer). This can be understood as an attempt to reduce the strain in the alliance by offering a general rationale for what he is doing. At the same time, it is a metacommunication about her tendency to fluctuate in terms of degree of openness. Since Joan's comments implicitly acknowledge some awareness of this, the therapist attempts to begin directing her attention to this process as it occurs in the moment.

T: Okay. Now is this "on topic" stuff?

J: I guess so.

T: Okay. You'll tell me when we get "off topic?"

J: Well, it's always hard to tell where things are gonna go. But at least you've stopped asking me how I felt about stuff when I complained about that . . . after a few times. Now, you finally believe me that I don't really feel things. (*Pause.*) Or else you're not letting on . . . you're accepting it and letting it go . . . that's probably closer to the truth.

T: (*Laughs.*)

J: I analyze everything. The other day I was talking to somebody and they said, "My goodness, you're thinking ahead all the time." 'Cause I had correctly anticipated everything that happened in our relationship.

T: It's true, my sense is that you do think ahead all the time. It's an important ability . . . but I imagine that it can also get kind of tiring sometimes.

J: Yeah . . . my mind's never at rest. I'm always on guard.

T: Do you have a sense of being on guard right now?

J: Yeah . . . somewhat . . .

T: What does it feel like to be on guard right now?

J: Well . . . it's like a wall is up.

T: How high is that wall right now?

J: Well, it's only part way up right now. It's not that high or thick.

Because of the ongoing tenuousness of the alliance and the shift in direction, the therapist once again explicitly negotiates agreement about the new therapeutic task. Joan makes it clear that she prefers this task to the task of exploring feelings and then speculates about what has led the therapist to become less persistent in his attempts to explore her feelings. Her speculations evoke a kind of narcissistic relish of her own analytic abilities. Perhaps this delight is partially defensive, motivated by a feeling of inadequacy in the moment about her own inability to explore feelings. The therapist joins with her by complimenting her on her analytic ability. He then offers an empathic conjecture about the negative side of the experience for her. This helps Joan to articulate her experience of always being on guard. The focus now returns to an in-the-moment exploration of fluctuations in Joan's degree of openness. In order to facilitate mindfulness, the therapist attempts to ground the exploration as much as possible in the here-and-now (e.g., "What does it feel like to be on guard right now?" and "How high is that wall right now?").

T: I'm going to suggest an experiment, if you're willing to try it.

J: Okay . . .

T: Can you think of the wall as a part of you, and give that part a voice?

J: How do you mean?

T: Actually speak as the wall. For example, "I'm Joan's wall, and this is what I do . . . etc."

J: Okay . . . I'm Joan's wall . . . I'm tough on the outside and don't let people in. I've got spikes and electric fences . . . and if anybody comes too close . . . zap!

T: Now . . . can you actually speak to me as the wall?

J: Okay . . . I won't let you touch me . . . because if you actually did touch me you might find a weak spot.

T: So it sounds like your wall is serving an important function.

J: Yeah . . . it's allowing me to live. It's allowing me not to turn into a jellyfish. (*Long pause.*)

T: What are you experiencing?

J: I don't know. I feel kind of strange ... kind of nervous. I never thought of it like that before.

Rather than conceptualizing the wall that Joan describes as a defense to be overcome, the therapist allies with the resistance, conceptualizing it as a part of the self that is not fully identified with. The focus is on awareness, not change. He attempts to give this aspect of the self a voice in the dialogue by suggesting an awareness experiment in which Joan speaks as the wall. This type of intervention can seem a little gimmicky, but it can also be a direct and powerful way of facilitating a new experientially grounded awareness. Despite her wariness, Joan takes to the experiment relatively easily. Identifying more fully with the self-protective function of the wall paradoxically helps her begin to access a more vulnerable aspect of the self (i.e., the experience of being like a jellyfish) that until now has been hidden from the therapist. This is a small but important shift that helps to lay the foundation for subsequent changes.

✳ 5

Stage-Process Models of Alliance Rupture Resolution

In this chapter, we outline two stage-process models that can be used to understand some of the characteristic ways in which ruptures in the therapeutic alliance are resolved in psychotherapy. Stage-process models are schemas that have been empirically developed to distill recurring patterns of change that take place across cases (Greenberg, 1986; Rice & Greenberg, 1984; Safran, Greenberg, & Rice, 1988). Psychotherapy process researchers have found that the development of such schemas provides a useful way of modeling important mechanisms of change in psychotherapy. The psychotherapy process can be seen as a sequence of recurring stages that take place in identifiable patterns. By identifying these stages and modeling patterns of transition between them, researchers have developed maps that can sensitize clinicians to sequential patterns that are likely to occur. The goal is not to offer rigidly prescriptive models, but rather to help clinicians develop pattern-recognition abilities that can facilitate the intervention process. We must emphasize that although these models do have heuristic value, they are oversimplifications of the complex processes that they attempt to capture.

The development of the models in this chapter (see Safran, Crocker, McMain, & Murray, 1990; Safran & Muran, 1996; Safran, Muran, & Samstag, 1994) is the product of more than a decade of research. This research has been guided by the task analytic paradigm for psychotherapy research developed by Leslie Greenberg and Laura Rice

(Greenberg, 1986; Rice & Greenberg, 1984; Safran, Greenberg, & Rice, 1988). This approach combines the rigorous analysis of single cases, using both qualitative and quantitative procedures, with model verification studies that test hypotheses about patterns of change, using aggregate data.

Following Heather Harper (1989a, 1989b), we have found it useful to organize ruptures into two subtypes: *withdrawal* and *confrontation*. In withdrawal ruptures, the patient withdraws or partially disengages from the therapist, his or her own emotions, or some aspect of the therapeutic process. Withdrawal ruptures can manifest in many different forms. In some cases, it is fairly obvious that the patient is having difficulty expressing his or her concerns or needs in the relationship—for example, a patient may express her concerns in an indirect or qualified way. In other cases, the patient complies or accommodates to the perceived desires of the therapist in such a subtle fashion that the therapist may have difficulty recognizing the patient's accommodation. It is not uncommon for therapists and patients to form a type of pseudoalliance that corresponds to the type of false self organization described by Winnicott (1960). In such cases, while therapeutic progress may take place at one level, therapy nevertheless perpetuates some self-defeating aspect of the patient's style. In confrontation ruptures, the patient directly expresses anger, resentment, or dissatisfaction with the therapist or with some aspect of the therapy. Table 5.1 (based on Harper's work) provides some examples of withdrawal and confrontation ruptures. Each rupture begins with a specific *marker* (Rice & Greenberg, 1984), a patient statement or action that signals the start of the rupture event.

Withdrawal and confrontation ruptures reflect patients' different ways of coping with the tension between their dialectically opposed needs for agency and relatedness. In withdrawal ruptures, patients strive for relatedness at the cost of the need for agency or self-definition. In confrontation ruptures, patients negotiate the conflict by favoring the need for agency or self-definition over the need for relatedness. Different patients are likely to present a predominance of one type of rupture over another; this predominance reflects different characteristic styles of coping or adaptation. Over the course of treatment, however, both types of ruptures may emerge with a specific patient, or both withdrawal and confrontation features may contribute to a specific impasse. Thus, it is critical for therapists to be sensitive to the specific qualities of the rupture that are emerging in the moment, rather than becoming locked into viewing patients as exclusively either confrontation or withdrawal types. In the following chapter, we elucidate the differences in resolving withdrawal and confrontation ruptures.

TABLE 5.1. Examples of Rupture Markers

Withdrawal	Confrontation Complaints about . . .
Denial (e.g., a patient denies a feeling state, such as anger, that was manifestly evident)	*Therapist as person* (e.g., a patient attacks the therapist's reserved manner as too passive)
Minimal response (e.g., a patient responds with short, clipped answers to open-ended, exploratory questions by the therapist)	*Therapist as competent* (e.g., a patient finds the therapist's comments useless and questions the therapist's skill)
Shifting the topic (e.g., a patient explores an issue and then suddenly shifts the focus onto something unrelated or remotely related)	*Activities of therapy* (e.g., a patient becomes irritated by the therapist's questions regarding internal feeling states and wonders aloud about their relevance)
Intellectualization (e.g., a patient discusses a painful experience in a detached, intellectualized manner)	*Being in therapy* (e.g., a patient confronts the therapist with doubts about continuing therapy)
Storytelling (e.g., a patient weaves overly elaborate stories or anecdotes to explain an experience)	*Parameters of therapy* (e.g., a patient complains about the inconvenience of the session time)
Talking about other (e.g., a patient spends an inordinate amount of time talking about other people and their doings)	*Progress in therapy* (e.g., a patient complains about the lack of significant gains in treatment)

The various stages of the models can be conceptualized as different tasks that are critical for the patient to engage in at different points in the resolution process, and as therapist interventions that can be facilitative. The patient tasks are not "tasks" in the sense of intentional actions, but rather in the sense of complex intrapsychic operations and interpersonal negotiations. The two models we outline are analogous to prototypes in Eleanor Rosch's (1988) sense. No one stage is critical to the resolution process, and the stages do not necessarily take place in the precise sequences predicted. These models do, however, tend to capture something essential about the resolution process in a probabilistic sense.

A RESOLUTION MODEL FOR WITHDRAWAL RUPTURES

The resolution model for withdrawal ruptures consists of five stages (see Figure 5.1). Each stage involves a particular patient task and spe-

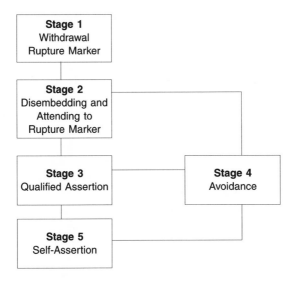

FIGURE 5.1. Rupture resolution model for withdrawal ruptures.

cific therapist interventions that we have observed to be facilitative. The specific interventions we describe in this chapter are not meant to constitute an exhaustive list; they are presented as examples.

Stage 1: Withdrawal Marker

The first stage is signaled by a patient *withdrawal marker*. For example, the patient complies with or defers to the therapist by agreeing with his interpretation in an acquiescent fashion. This type of withdrawal is often part of an ongoing enactment in which the therapist becomes embedded in the patient's relational matrix and responds to the patient's passive or submissive behavior by brushing over any subtle indications of concern or by acting in an overly directive or domineering fashion. For example, the patient responds to an interpretation in an acquiescent fashion, and the therapist continues to elaborate on his interpretation. In Core Conflictual Relationship Theme (CCRT) terms, the patient withdrawal marker can be conceptualized as a *response of self*, a characteristic way of responding in anticipation of not having an underlying wish fulfilled. The therapist's embedded actions can be conceptualized as a *response of other*.

Stage 2: Disembedding and Attending to the Rupture Marker

In this stage, therapists begin drawing attention to the rupture and establishing a focus on the here-and-now of the therapeutic relationship. To the extent that they are embedded in the patient's relational matrix at this point, they will need to begin to develop some awareness of the nature of their participation in it. Although for heuristic purposes we are discussing this disembedding process as if it is one discrete step in a linear pathway, it is important to bear in mind that the process of disembedding is never complete. Over the course of the resolution process, therapist and patient cycle back and forth between greater and lesser degrees of embeddedness.

In those situations in which the withdrawal marker is particularly subtle, the therapist's awareness of his or her own feelings or action tendencies may be the best indicator that something is taking place that warrants exploration. For example, therapists may find themselves working harder than usual to give advice to a patient, being less attentive to a patient's concerns than they typically would be with other patients, ignoring a patient's concerns, or pushing a patient to accept an interpretation or to look at things in a certain way. In situations in which the patient withdraws by dissociating threatening feelings about the therapist, therapists may find themselves suddenly losing interest in the patient or becoming aware that their attention has been drifting.

Once the therapist begins to become aware of the cycle being enacted, his or her tasks are to disembed from it and to begin to explore the feelings that are being avoided by the patient. These two processes are interdependent. For example, a therapist who becomes aware of her attention drifting may begin to metacommunicate by disclosing this experience to her patient and probing for his experience. The therapist might say: "I'm aware of my attention wandering. I'm not sure what's going on, but I think it may have something to do with a kind of distant sound in your voice. Any sense of what's going on for you right now?" In response, the patient is able to acknowledge that he is withdrawing from the therapist because he feels hurt by something she said.

During this stage, it is important to direct the patient's attention to the here-and-now of the therapeutic relationship. Useful interventions consist of statements such as "What are you experiencing?" or "I have a sense of you withdrawing from me" or "How are you feeling about what's going on between us right now?"

It is critical for the therapist to maintain a curious, empathic stance toward the patient and to be open and receptive to any negative feelings that begin to emerge. It is common at this point for patients to speak about negative feelings in general terms, rather than directly confronting the therapist. For example, the patient may complain about the mental health profession in general. In response, the therapist may find it useful to explore the relevance of these feelings to the present situation. For example, the therapist might say: "If you're willing, I'd like to ask you to experiment with personalizing what you're saying. Do these concerns apply to me as well?"

This exploration should be conducted in a noncontrolling fashion, one that respects any decision on the patient's part not to discuss negative feelings toward the therapist in the present context. This is particularly important with patients who tend to be compliant; to push for something the patient is not ready to explore simply invites more compliance. Therapists should be mindful of the possibility of contributing to a new variation of an enactment through their attempts to reestablish contact with patients who are withdrawing. Any intervention can be made in the service of perpetuating an ongoing enactment.

Although we have highlighted the role of the therapist in the process of disembedding, we by no means intend to portray this process as a one-sided enterprise. It invariably includes the patient's willingness to participate in a process of collaborative inquiry about the nature of the interactive matrix. In some way, the patient must also be willing and able to step out of the enactment in order to begin an exploration of what is going on in the therapeutic relationship.

The disembedding stage is followed by two parallel pathways of exploration. The first is termed the *Experiencing Pathway*. This involves the exploration of thoughts and feelings associated with the rupture (Stages 3 and 5). The second, referred to as the *Avoidance Pathway*, involves the exploration of internal processes and defensive operations that interfere or interrupt feelings and thoughts associated with the rupture experience (Stage 4). The *Experiencing Pathway* can be subdivided into two successive stages: Stage 3 (*Qualified Assertion*) and Stage 5 (*Assertion*).

Stage 3: Qualified Assertion

In the *Qualified Assertion* stage, the patient begins to express thoughts and feelings associated with the rupture experience. These, however, are mixed with features of the initial rupture marker. For example, the patient begins to express negative sentiments, but then qualifies the negative statement or takes it back (e.g., "I'm feeling a little irritated, but it's not a big deal"). In this stage, the patient comes closer to contacting and expressing underlying wishes that are typically self-assertive in nature and are often associated with angry feelings. Such content becomes too anxiety-provoking, however, and the patient ultimately withdraws from full acknowledgment and experience of those feelings.

A number of therapist interventions can be helpful in the context of this type of qualified assertion. These are grouped together under the general rubric of *facilitating assertion*. The most important principle here is to empathize with and display a genuine interest and curiosity in the negative sentiments that are expressed. One intervention involves *differentiating and exploring different self-states*. When the patient qualifies his statements or indicates that he is uncertain or conflicted about his negative feelings, the therapist can acknowledge both sides and then focus selectively on the concerns that the patient is having difficulty acknowledging or articulating. For example, the therapist might say: "I understand that you're uncertain about how important your concerns are. If you're willing to go into it, however, I'd be interested in hearing more." Or she might say: "It sounds like you have two perspectives on this issue. One part of you feels that it's no big deal, but the other part has some concerns. If you're willing to pursue this a little further, I'm going to suggest that you try putting the part that feels 'It's no big deal' aside for a moment, and let me hear more from the part that's concerned."

Another useful intervention consists of *providing the patient with feedback* about the way in which she qualifies or softens her statement in order to heighten her awareness of this process. For example, the therapist might remark: "My sense is that you start to express some negative feelings, but then you end up pulling your punch. Do you have any awareness of this?" If the patient is able to become more aware of this defensive operation, the therapist can begin to explore the internal processes associated with this avoidance. For example, the therapist might ask: "Any sense of what the risk would be of putting things in an unqualified way?"

A third intervention consists of suggesting an *awareness experiment*. This involves encouraging the patient to experiment with directly expressing feelings that the therapist hypothesizes are being avoided and then to attend to whatever feelings are evoked by the experiment. In some cases, the experiment evokes anxiety, which can then lead to an exploration of the internal processes associated with the avoidance. For example, a patient says: "I'm feeling a little frustrated with the pace at which things are moving, but I know that there's no magic pill." The therapist then responds: "I'm wondering if you're willing to try saying something as an experiment. Try saying, 'I want more from you' and see how it feels." The patient responds: "I can't say that." The therapist then asks: "Why not? What happens for you when you think of saying it?" The patient then responds: "I start to feel childish." This admission subsequently leads to an exploration of the patient's harsh and condemning attitude toward his own needs. In other cases, the experiment helps to deepen the patient's awareness and acknowledgment of the avoided experience. In the above illustration, the patient might, for example, repeat the phrase "I want more from you" or some variant of it; then, when the therapist asks, "What do you experience as you say that?," the patient contacts some of his disowned yearning.

Stage 4: Avoidance

In a typical resolution process, the exploration of the rupture *Experiencing Pathway* proceeds to a certain point and then becomes blocked. The blockage is indicated by the patient engaging in coping strategies, defensive verbalizations and actions that function to avoid or manage the emotions associated with the rupture experience. Examples of coping strategies include changing the topic, speaking in a deadened voice tone, and speaking in general terms rather than the here-and-now specifics of the therapeutic relationship. The *Avoidance Pathway* involves the exploration of beliefs, expectations, and other internal processes that inhibit the acknowledgment and expression of feelings and needs associated with the rupture experience.

There are two major subtypes here. The first consists of *beliefs and expectations about the other's response* that interfere with the exploration of the Experiencing Pathway. In CCRT terms, these are conceptualized as the patient's *expected response of other*. For example, the patient who expects expressions of anger to evoke retaliation will have difficulty acknowledging and expressing angry feelings, while the patient who believes that expressions of vulnerability and need will result in abandonment will have difficulty expressing such feelings. The therapist responses that are most facilitative in this context are *exploration and sustained empathy*. Let's suppose the patient speaks critically about therapists in general, but has difficulty being directly critical of his own therapist. The therapist could respond: "I'm aware of you speaking about therapists in general, but not specifically about me. Any sense of what the risk would be of speaking specifically about me?" In another example, the patient begins to ask the therapist to be more helpful and then qualifies his request (e.g., "It's not a big deal"). The therapist responds: "I'm aware of you qualifying or softening your request. Any sense of what makes it difficult to ask without qualifying?"

Explorations of this type are best conducted as close as possible to the moment in which the avoidance has taken place. Moreover, they should be phrased in a way that encourages patients to discover their experience in the moment (e.g., "I'm afraid of offending you"), rather than to engage in intellectually distant speculation (e.g., "It relates to my fear of authority figures"). A sustained empathic stance by the therapist is critical at this point. It is important for the therapist not to challenge the patient's fears in any way since this will only make it difficult for him or her to articulate them more fully. Without such articulation, the patient will lose the opportunity of evaluating his or her fears in more detail in light of the therapist's actual actions.

The second subtype of avoidance consists of *self-doubts or self-criticisms*, which function to block the exploration of the rupture *Experiencing Pathway*. For example, the patient who believes she is childish for wanting help will not be able to express her needs to the therapist, or the patient who believes that she is immature for being angry will have difficulty expressing those angry feelings to the therapist. This type of self-criticism can be understood developmentally as an introject or negative responses of the other that have been internalized. In CCRT terms, they would be conceptualized as internal *responses of self*. A common mistake therapists make at this point is to view the self-doubt or criticism in this context as a mark of progress, rather than as a sign of avoidance. This is particularly likely to happen when therapists are feeling threatened by the negative feelings or wishes that their patients are avoiding.

In general, it is useful for the therapist to help the patient to *differentiate and explore different self-states* in this context. The therapist can draw the patient's attention to the way in which she shifts into a state of self-criticism when she begins to contact self-assertive feelings and help her to frame her experience as a conflict between two different parts of the self. He can then ask the patient to speak directly from each aspect of the self, alternating between the part of the self that wishes to assert itself and the part of the self that criticizes that wish. In this way, a dialogue can be established between the two aspects of the self that allows the patient to ultimately come to have a tangible experience of the way in which she interferes with her own desire to assert.

As patients explore their avoidance, gain awareness of the processes interfering with their experience, and develop more of a sense of ownership of these processes, feelings associated with the rupture experience naturally begin to emerge more fully. Patients may move back to the *Experiencing Pathway* spontaneously, or therapists may redirect attention to it once again. Typically, a resolution process involves an ongoing alternation between *Experiencing* and *Avoidance Pathways*, with the exploration of each pathway functioning to facilitate a deepening of the exploration of the other.

Stage 5: Self-Assertion

In Stage 5, the patient accesses and *expresses underlying needs* to the therapist. In CCRT terms, this act of self-assertion would be conceptualized as the expression of the underlying *wish*. It can sometimes be difficult for therapists to distinguish between this type of self-assertion and the preliminary assertion that takes place in Stage 3. Self-assertion in this context entails an acceptance of responsibility for one's needs and desires, rather than an expectation that the other will automatically know what one needs or that he or she is obligated to fulfill them. It thus implies a certain degree of patient individuation with respect to the therapist. In contrast, the expression of wishes and needs in Stage 3 often has a pleading, apologetic, or demanding tone. It is mediated by the patient's self-criticism or expectation that his or her needs will not be met. It is thus more akin to the expression of neediness than to the expression of need (Ghent, 1992, 1993).

Once the patient has begun to assert herself and express an underlying wish, it is important for the therapist to respond in an empathic and nonjudgmental way. This kind of response plays an important role in challenging the expectations (both conscious and unconscious) that have made it difficult for the patient to self-assert in the first place. A common pattern is for patients to initially assert themselves in a manner that is structured by their characteristic relational schema—for example, a patient whose father was tyrannical and critical, asks the therapist to be more confrontative. When a patient asserts in this manner, the therapist should try to empathize with the patient's desire, rather than to immediately interpret it as a reflection of an old relational schema. The latter response risks discouraging patients from asserting themselves more and can lead them to further submerge their underlying wishes. In contrast, when therapists empathize with their patients' desires, it helps them to assert themselves in a fashion that is less structured by their old schema. Thus, the patient in the above example may ultimately be able to ask the therapist to be more supportive.

Clinical Illustration

In order to further clarify the withdrawal resolution model outlined in Figure 5.1, we illustrate it with the following transcript from the fifth session of a treatment:

> The patient, Lisa, was a 32-year-old woman who sought treatment because of a general lack of direction in her life and her specific difficulty finding and sustaining a long-term romantic relationship with a man. She had a history of abandonment: her father abandoned the family when she was 8, and her mother died of cancer when she was in her teens. The patient and her younger sister had subsequently been raised by an aunt who had never married. While her sister married in her early 20s, Lisa was still unmarried and continued to live with her aunt. The patient begins the fifth session by announcing that her schedule at work is in flux, so that it will be difficult to set up a regular appointment.

Stage 1: Withdrawal Marker

LISA (L): It's going to be difficult.

THERAPIST (T): You mean your schedule will be continuously changing?

L: Umm . . . that's right.

T: I can see how that would be a problem.

L: Got anything by correspondence? (*Laughs.*)

T: No.

L: Any good books to read? I don't know what else to do. All I can do is play it by ear and see when I'm able to . . . when I'm in the area or something, if we can work it that way.

T: So you're thinking perhaps . . . if it turns out you're free sometime you could drop in?

L: Yeah . . . can you do it that way?

T: Uh . . . no. I don't think that would be very useful.

L: Well, can you think of anything else that would be useful?

T: I'm not really sure what to suggest. What kind of thing do you have in mind?

L: I don't know. I'm just asking you. I thought maybe you had a broader knowledge of what's happening out there. Something that could fit with my needs.

T: There are people around who have hours in the evenings. Maybe the best thing to do would be to look into that. [Lisa was being seen in a free clinic with only daytime hours.]

L: Can you suggest any names for me?

T: I can probably come up with one or two.

L: Other than that, I would just have to call around myself?

T: I suppose.

L: I don't know. There's always a dilemma. Something always comes around and screws things up.

Stage 2: Disembedding and Attending to the Rupture

T: I guess I'm a little curious and kind of taken by surprise, because when we started you were aware that you were going to be starting a new job.

L: Yeah, but I didn't know exactly what my schedule would be.

T: Anything else going on for you?

L: No, that's about it. What would you do if you were in my situation?

T: I'm not sure, to be frank.

L: Well, I'm only doing what's right . . . right for me, anyway.

T: I'm wondering what's going on for you inside?

L: I'm wondering what you're thinking?

T: I guess I'm aware of feeling like I'm being kind of withholding with you. Does that fit with your experience at all?

L: Yeah, I guess, a little.

T: Can you say anymore?

L: Well, I'm not sure if you're really giving me what I need. Maybe that was true last session as well.

Rather than directly acknowledging her frustration with the last session, Lisa begins this session by indicating that her job schedule may make it difficult to make future appointments. She does not directly say that she wants to terminate treatment, but she does imply that she may terminate (e.g., asking about therapy by correspondence or relevant books) and then asks the therapist if he can accommodate to her erratic schedule. When the therapist rules out this possibility, she continues to seek direction from the therapist in terms of a possible referral. The therapist appears to be embedded in an enactment in which he responds to Lisa's unstated anger and ongoing requests for accommodation and guidance with irritation and withholdingness. He finally articulates his sense that he is being withholding, thereby beginning the process of disembedding. This helps Lisa to begin to more directly acknowledge her frustration.

Stage 4: Avoidance

L: But then I think, "Maybe I'm not really giving things a chance." That happens to me all the time. I always question myself.

T: So you start to feel frustrated, but then it sounds like you start to question yourself.

L: Yeah.

T: It sounds like there are two sides of you caught in a little bit of a struggle. Does that make sense?

L: Yeah.

Stage 3: Qualified Assertion

T: Which of these two are you feeling more strongly right now?

L: A little frustrated . . . but maybe I'm being demanding.

T: Are you open to exploring your frustration a little more?

Stage 4: Avoidance

L: I don't know.

T: Any sense of what your reservations are?

L: Well, I wouldn't want to say something that you took the wrong way.

T: What might happen if I took it the wrong way?

L: I don't know. . . . You might take it personally.

T: And what if I took it personally?

L: I might hurt your feelings (*long pause and Lisa looks pensive*).

T: Any sense of what you're experiencing right now?

This segment alternates back and forth between the exploration of the avoidance and the experience. After beginning to express her frustration, Lisa begins to doubt herself. The therapist intervenes simply by labeling the two different self-states (experiencing vs. self-doubting) and by beginning to explore the state that emerges as more figural in the moment (frustration). This evokes anxiety and further avoidance on Lisa's part, which is subsequently explored in greater depth. Through this process, Lisa is able to articulate her fear of hurting the therapist if she were to directly express her negative sentiments.

Stage 5: Self-Assertion

L: . . . Maybe a little angry.

T: Uh-huh, can you put some of your feelings into words?

L: Why should I have to worry about *your* feelings? I don't see any progress. I guess I want to know what's going to make me function better. Like I want you to tell me what it is about me that stops me from being a functioning person. Why is it that I'm always getting into these predicaments? I guess I want you to tell me what to do.

T: Okay. So I'm going to see if I'm understanding what you're saying.

L: Okay.

T: You can tell me whether or not I've got it. You're saying, "I want to know what's going on ... what's blocking me from doing what I want to do, or from being more happy and contented."

L: Yeah.

T: And sort of "I want you to tell me or show me in a way" ... something like that. Can you say a little more?

L: Basically, I want to hear what you have to say. I mean I've given you the facts, and I guess you know what my insights are ... I guess I want you to wrap it up and tell me what you think. (*At this point, she makes an emphatic gesture with her hand.*)

T: (*The therapist mirrors the gesture.*) When you make that gesture, what kind of feeling goes with it?

L: I don't know. It's like ... "It's your show" or something.

T: "It's your show?"

L: Yeah ... you know ... the ball's in your court.

T: Okay ... "The ball's in your court." It sounds like it feels like I keep putting the ball back in your court, rather than really taking responsibility for helping you.

L: Yeah ... I guess that's it.

T: What are you experiencing?

The process of explicitly articulating her fear of hurting the therapist's feelings spontaneously helps Lisa to contact her anger at sacrificing her own needs. In response to the therapist's empathy and probing, she is finally able to explicitly articulate the demand that has been implicit in her communication so far. By drawing attention to Lisa's hand gesture, the therapist helps her to further articulate her demand ("It's your show" and "The ball's in your court"). The therapist then empathizes with the experience underlying this demand ("It sounds like I keep putting the ball back in your court rather than really taking responsibility for helping you").

Stage 4: Avoidance

L: I feel shy.

T: What's your shyness about?

L: Well ... it seems a little bit ridiculous. It's almost like admitting I'm defeated and asking for help.

T: Asking for help?

L: Uh-huh . . . Just like when you're a kid. Going and asking people for directions or something. You're a little hesitant, a little shy maybe, you know, insecure about it. Why should they help you?

The therapist's empathic statement appears to have evoked some experience in Lisa of the unmet need underlying the demand, and consequent anxiety and self-recrimination. In response to the therapist's probes, she is also able to begin articulating a fear of abandonment (although a detailed exploration of this fear in relationship to the therapist awaited later sessions). After this session, Lisa recommitted herself to the treatment, and her work schedule never reemerged as an issue.

Although in many withdrawal ruptures expressing negative feelings that have been unacknowledged about the therapy or therapeutic process constitutes the final stage of the resolution process, this example ends with a preliminary exploration of the patient's disavowed needs for nurturance. This theme emerged as one particularly important for Lisa, whose expectations of abandonment played an important role in perpetuating a vacillation between resentful compliance and indirect demands for nurturance. Although her angry demandingness emerged as a secondary reaction to an underlying wish for nurturance, the direct expression of this demand nevertheless constituted an important act of self-assertion in the context of this resolution process, since it enabled her to begin to take responsibility for her demands, rather than expressing them indirectly.

A RESOLUTION MODEL
FOR CONFRONTATION RUPTURES

Confrontation ruptures are likely to arouse intense and disturbing feelings of anger, impotence, self-indictment, and even despair in therapists. While such feelings are a common response to withdrawal ruptures as well, therapists often find being the object of intense aggression for a prolonged period of time particularly difficult to deal with. In the face of such intense and disturbing feelings, it is critical to remember that what is most important is not the specific therapeutic interventions employed, but rather the whole process of surviving. As we discussed in Chapter 3, tolerating patients' critical and angry feelings is a difficult task. It is inevitable that therapists will respond as human beings with their own anger and defensiveness. Nonetheless, therapists must stay mindful and aware of the difficult feelings that are emerging in them as they experience themselves as objects of their patients' aggression, and they must be willing to acknowledge their contributions to the interaction on an ongoing basis. Their task in this context is not to avoid or to transcend angry or defensive feelings, but to demonstrate a consistent willingness to stick with the patient and to work toward understanding what is going on between them in the face of whatever difficult feelings emerge for both of them.

The resolution model for confrontation ruptures in many ways resembles the resolution model for withdrawal markers. It begins with the rupture marker in Stage 1 and continues with the disembedding process in Stage 2. It also includes the two parallel pathways of exploration: the *Experiencing Pathway* and the *Avoidance Pathway*. It differs, however, in a number of respects. First, to the extent that patients present with intense aggression, the processes of disembedding from and surviving the patient's aggression over an extended period of time become more central. Second, the emphasis in Stage 3 is on elucidating patients' construal of the situation, rather than on helping them begin to assert themselves and individuate. For example, the patient may begin to put into words the way in which he feels let down and disappointed by the therapist. Third, the wishes and needs emerging in the final stage typically entail a desire for contact or nurturance rather than a desire for individuation. Fourth, we make a distinction between patients' avoidance of aggression (Stage 4) and their avoidance of vulnerable feelings (Stage 5).

In CCRT terms, a confrontation marker can be conceptualized as an aggressive *response of self* that is perpetuated by a vicious cycle in which the patient believes her *wish* for nurturance will continue to go unmet; that others will respond with abandonment, impingement, or retaliation; and that the only hope for survival and possible remediation of the situation consists of self-protection and attempts to coerce the other into meeting her needs. Thus, in Ghent's (1992) terms, the therapist is presented with an expression of neediness that covers an underlying need. As Figure 5.2 illustrates, the common progression in the resolution of confrontation ruptures consists of moving through *feelings of anger* (Stage 1), *to underlying feelings of injury, disappointment, or hurt* (Stage 3), *to contacting vulnerability and underlying wishes for nurturance* (Stage 6).

Stage 1: Confrontation Marker

Confrontation ruptures typically begin as some variant of the patient's habitual *response of self*. For example, a patient has a long-thwarted desire to be nurtured or taken care of and a readiness to perceive the therapist as one more in a long line of people who will fail him. He

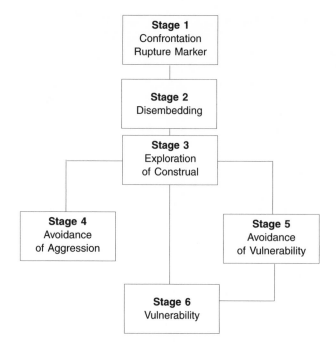

FIGURE 5.2. Rupture resolution model for confrontation ruptures.

thus enters into the therapeutic relationship with a reservoir of disappointment and rage waiting to be triggered by the therapist's inevitable failings and shortcomings. When confrontation ruptures take place, it can be difficult, if not impossible, for therapists to avoid responding to the patient's demands or criticisms defensively, thereby providing the *expected response of other*. As Henry, Schacht, and Strupp (1986) have shown, it is all too common for therapist interpretations to subtly convey blaming and belittling messages to their patients, or to consist of complex communications that simultaneously convey helping *and* critical messages.

Stage 2: Disembedding

When this takes place, the process of exploring the interactive matrix becomes the therapist's priority. The therapist's first step in working through a confrontation rupture involves disembedding from the vicious cycle of hostility and counterhostility that is being enacted by metacommunicating to the patient about the current struggle. As we discussed in the context of withdrawal ruptures, although we are representing disembedding as a distinct stage, the entire resolution process involves an ongoing cycling back and forth between greater and lesser degrees of embeddedness. During the disembedding process, it is often critical for therapists to acknowledge responsibility for *their* contribution to the interaction. For example, the therapist might say: "I think that what's been going on is that I've been feeling criticized by you and have responded by trying to blame you for what's going on in our interaction." It can also be extremely useful in this context for therapists to comment on the experience of a mutual struggle. For example, the therapist could declare: "It feels to me like you and I are in a power struggle right now, with me trying to hold you responsible for your frustrations with therapy, and you trying to pin the blame on me."

Therapists who feel pressured to prove to the patient that therapy will be helpful can comment on their dilemma, rather than responding to this pressure either with ineffectual attempts at persuasion or with angry defensiveness. For example, the therapist might remark: "I'm feeling pressured to convince you that I can help you, but I have a feeling that nothing I say will seem compelling to you." Therapists who feel criticized or attacked can comment on this experience rather than defending themselves or counterattacking. For example, the therapist might say: "I feel wary of saying anything because I feel criticized when I try to respond to your questions or concerns." This type of metacommunication can serve a number of functions. First, it can help the therapist to reestablish internal space that has collapsed. Second, it can provide the patient with feedback that can help him to acknowledge negative feelings toward the therapist that are disowned. Third, it can help patients to stand behind their actions.

1. *Reestablishing internal space.* When therapists are the objects of intense aggression, they can become paralyzed by their own internal conflicts concerning their aggressive feelings, and this can make it impossible for them to reflect more fully on what is taking place in the interaction. Under such circumstances, it is inevitable that there will be a collapsing of *internal space*, or analytic space, that is, the type of double consciousness necessary to be a participant-observer. The simple process of articulating aspects of their experience that feel threatening in this context—"saying the unsayable"—can begin the process of freeing therapists up and restoring analytic space. Such articulation does not involve discharging hostile feelings toward patients; rather, the therapist should attempt to selectively articulate aspects of his experience of the situation in as tactful a fashion as possible. Often it is useful for therapists to convey some sense of their own feelings of conflict around the situation. For example, the therapist might disclose: "I'm

feeling really attacked and am struggling not to respond defensively" or "I'm reluctant to say anything for fear of provoking another attack from you" or "I'm feeling attacked and kind of angry, but afraid to show my anger for fear of escalating things between us."

2. *Providing the patient with feedback.* Providing aggressive patients with feedback about their impact can help them begin to see their contribution to the interaction. We agree with theorists such as Carpy (1989), Epstein (1977), and Gabbard (1996) that attempts to interpret patients' anger in this context as a reflection of an internal dynamic, such as projected aggression, can be deleterious to the therapeutic process. This type of interpretation implies that the anger resides *only* in the patient, *not* in the therapist, and as such it can function as a way of expressing therapists' angry feelings in a disavowed fashion. Providing feedback of the type described above, however, neither blames patients for the interaction nor pretends to place therapists outside the interaction, poised on some type of neutral therapeutic perch. Moreover, when therapists struggle with the process of articulating selected aspects of their painful and conflicting feelings about an aggressive interaction, the effort itself conveys to patients the healthy message that aggressive feelings are not too toxic to be talked about and dealt with explicitly. This can ultimately help them to feel more comfortable about fully acknowledging their own angry feelings.

3. *Helping patients to stand behind their actions.* Confrontation ruptures occur on a continuum in terms of how directly or indirectly the initial confrontation is expressed. When the initial confrontation takes place in a more direct fashion, the therapist does not need to begin by facilitating a more direct expression of the underlying demand or negative sentiments. In many cases, however, the initial confrontation is mixed with features of a withdrawal marker. When this takes place, therapists may become embedded in an enactment that is particularly difficult to see because patients are communicating in a complex and incongruent fashion. For example, a patient may complain about the therapy, but at the same time deny that he is unhappy with things as they are. When this happens, the therapist's first task, as part of the process of disembedding, is to attempt to clarify the nature of the incongruent communication that is taking place. This clarification process involves helping patients to express the underlying negative feelings more directly, thereby standing behind their actions. For example, the first step in working with a patient who is sarcastically expressing her negative feelings toward the therapist, but at the same time acting in a conciliatory fashion, is to help her to acknowledge the angry feelings underlying the sarcasm and to express them directly.

The first step in working with the patient who is *implicitly* making demands of the therapist is to help him to make the demands more *explicitly*. A useful intervention to facilitate this process is for therapists to disclose the impact the patient is having on them. For example, the therapist might say: "I feel attacked and protected at the same time" or "It feels to me like you, in a somewhat cautious way, are trying to get me to do more for you." As in the case with the withdrawal model, interventions of this type can lead either to an exploration of *the experience associated with the rupture* or *the avoidance of that experience*. And as is also the case with the withdrawal model, this phase of the resolution process typically involves an oscillation back and forth between the *Experiencing* and *Avoidance Pathways*.

The transition towards the *Exploration of Construal* (Stage 3) is facilitated through a number of processes that take place in the *Disembedding* Stage. For example:

1. By metacommunicating about the interaction, rather than simply retaliating or withdrawing, therapists can begin the process of articulating what is actually going on in the interaction and exploring patients' construal of it. For example, the therapist says: "I have a sense that anything I say strikes you the wrong way right now. Does that fit with your experience?" The patient tentatively acknowledges that it does, and the therapist then asks her to elaborate on the experience of having everything the therapist says strike her the wrong way. Or a patient demands an explanation of how therapy works, and the therapist responds: "Although I feel it's important to answer your question, I have a sense that nothing I say will be acceptable to you. Does that fit with your experience in any way?" In response, the patient acknowledges there may be something to the therapist's perception. Further probing subsequently helps the patient articulate the construal associated with finding nothing acceptable (e.g., a sense of futility and hopelessness).

2. By acknowledging patients' impact on them, including whatever vulnerable or impotent feelings they may have, therapists can deescalate the attack and pave the way for exploring the construal underlying it.

3. When patients confront therapists in an indirect fashion, therapists should help them to confront more directly. In this way, they will develop a greater awareness of the feelings motivating the confrontation, thereby facilitating access to the underlying construal processes.

4. Sometimes therapists' ability to express their own feelings of anger in a reflective fashion or to acknowledge their own conflicts around their feelings can help to establish them as real subjects for patients, rather than as objects. Moreover, in contrast to therapists' at-

tempts to interpret patients' anger or to hide their own disturbing feelings, this type of acknowledgment can help patients to experience their own potency, thereby giving them the necessary security to begin exploring their underlying construal. In addition, by expressing their own negative and aggressive feelings in a modulated fashion, therapists can play an important role in detoxifying patients' own aggression for them by providing a model of the way in which aggression can be processed without being catastrophic (Carpy, 1991; Weiss et al., 1986; Winnicott, 1965).

5. When therapists acknowledge their own contribution to the interaction, it can decrease the experience that patients may have of feeling persecuted or assaulted. As a result, they may feel less of a need to protect themselves by attacking, thereby allowing them to begin exploring their construal of the situation in a more differentiated way.

Stage 3: Exploration of Construal

The therapist's task in Stage 3 is to help patients begin to unpack their construal of the interaction. For example, a patient experiences the therapist as patronizing him or as blaming him for the fact that the treatment is not progressing more quickly, or a patient experiences the therapist as withholding and as not providing needed direction. The therapist's task here is to elucidate the nuances of the patient's perceptions (which are often associated with feelings of anger, injury, or disappointment). This process of unpacking involves a phenomenological exploration of patients' conscious experience and an articulation of that which is on the edge of awareness, but not fully explicit. It does not involve interpretations that require inferences about unconscious dynamics.

As we discussed earlier, interpretations of patients' anger in terms of disowned aggression or envy are usually not helpful at this stage. Similarly, attempts to bypass patients' anger by interpreting it as a response to underlying need or vulnerability are usually nonproductive. As contemporary ego analysts, such as Gray (1994) and Busch (1995), suggest, attempting to bypass the patient's conscious experience in this fashion can be experienced by the patient as unempathic and disempowering. Moreover, such an attempt may in part be motivated by therapists' attempts to take themselves out of the line of fire and to put themselves back in control. It is important for patients to experience any feelings of anger, hurt, or disappointment that exist as valid, acceptable, and tolerable, before they can begin to explore primary yearnings that are more vulnerable in nature. The acknowledgment of underlying needs of a more vulnerable type must emerge in an organic fashion out of the therapeutic relationship as the patient and therapist struggle together to work through whatever aggressive cycle is being enacted.

When therapists are able to become aware of their own contribution to the interactive matrix, it can be useful to acknowledge this contribution openly. When they cannot initially see their own contribution to the situation, they should encourage patients to articulate their perception of how the therapist has contributed (Aron, 1996). In this process, it is critical for therapists to be open to learning something new about themselves and their contributions to the interaction, rather than to think of this process exclusively as a way of exploring patients' underlying construal processes. This openness can transform the situation by reducing patients' need to be defensive and by making it easier for them to verbalize subtle perceptions that may be difficult to fully articulate in the absence of a receptive audience.

For example, in one case where the patient felt his therapist was insensitive and callous in rearranging an appointment time, it was critical for the therapist to be open to acknowledging this possibility in order to facilitate the exploration of the patient's concern that the therapist did not care for him. This led into an exploration of the patient's general mistrust of people's caring. In another case where the therapist had recently given birth, it was critical for her to listen and learn about the ways in which she had changed in her manner toward the patient before the patient could contact and explore fears regarding the emotional availability of others. As patients articulate the nuances of their perceptions, therapists begin to understand them from an internal point of reference. When this happens, they are less likely to take things personally and less likely to respond defensively. At the same time, patients begin to feel understood and validated, and some of their pent-up fury and rage begins to dissipate.

In some cases, the therapist's ability to help the patient unpack her construal and to empathize with her experience constitutes the end of the resolution process. In other cases, things proceed to a deeper exploration of underlying wishes of a more vulnerable nature (Stage 6), a process we will discuss below.

Stage 4: Avoidance of Aggression

During Stages 2 (*Disembedding*) and 3 (*Exploration of Construal*), it is important for therapists to monitor subtle shifts in the patient's self-states on an ongoing basis (see Chapter 2). Even those patients who are most overtly aggressive or hostile toward their therapists will experience moments of anxiety or guilt about the expression of such aggressive feelings and attempt to undo the harm they feel they have done by justifying their actions or attempting to depersonalize the situation in order to defuse the felt danger.

If therapists are feeling too overwhelmed by their own emotional response to patients' aggression, they may have difficulty tracking these shifts. Consequently, they will miss an important opportunity to explore a habitual mode of patient functioning. For example, patients may cycle back and forth between a state of anger at the therapist, guilt over their expression of aggression, and a state of anger triggered by the feelings of guilt that are experienced as intolerable (Horowitz, 1987). In this type of situation, it can be very useful for therapists to track these subtle shifts in self-states and to help patients become aware of the internal processes that lead to these shifts.

Stage 5: Avoidance of Vulnerability

A second type of avoidance that sometimes emerges during the resolution of confrontation ruptures consists of the defensive withdrawal from vulnerable feelings. In some situations, patients will begin to contact vulnerable feelings and then shift back into a more familiar and secure state of aggression. When this happens, it can be useful for the therapist to track the shift and attempt to draw the patient's attention to it. For example, the therapist might note: "My sense is that you began to contact some sadness there and then suddenly shifted into a harder or more aggressive stance. Did you have any awareness of this?" If the patient is able to become aware of the shift, the therapist can then explore his or her internal processes. For example, the therapist might ask: "Any sense of what went on inside just before the shift took place?" At first, patients will often have difficulty becoming aware of this type of shift. Even when they do become more aware, they will continue to have difficulty identifying relevant internal triggers. Over time, however, they can develop some facility at tracking their own shifts in self-state and can begin to explore internal processes triggering the shift (e.g., fears of abandonment or self-criticism for being vulnerable).

Stage 6: Vulnerability

Primary needs and wishes underlying the patient's aggression may take a long time (months or years) to emerge; in some more extreme cases, they may never emerge. When the therapist has demonstrated consistently over an extended period of time a willingness to take the concerns underlying the patient's aggression seriously, an attempt to understand them from the patient's internal point of reference, a willingness to explore and acknowledge his or her own contribution to the interaction, and an ability to survive the patient's aggression, it paves the way for vulnerable feelings and wishes that have been defended against to emerge. When they do emerge, it is often initially in the form of an acknowledgment of despair.

In contrast to earlier stages of the resolution process, however, in which despair may emerge in a cynical, angry fashion that pushes others away, by now the relationship has evolved to the point that there is something different about both patient and therapist. Over time the patient has come to trust the therapist to the point where she can begin to let him in on the pain and sadness associated with her despair, and the therapist has evolved to the point where he has a deeper appreciation of the patient as a whole person and is better able to empathize with her despair.

As we discussed in Chapter 2, the experience of having the therapist care for her in her pain and despair can be an important new experience for the patient—one that allows her for the first time to escape her feeling of isolation and to begin to have more compassion for herself. This in turn facilitates the emergence of underlying needs for nurturance that have been disowned. It is critical for therapists to respond to any primary and more vulnerable feeling states that emerge in this context in an empathic and validating way. It is important not to view these feelings as archaic infantile needs that must be understood and renounced, or even as remobilized development yearnings, but rather as normal human yearnings for nurturance and support.

In some cases, it can be important for therapists to gratify the patient's wish. For example, a patient who had traditionally had a tremendous amount of difficulty acknowledging and expressing underlying needs eventually came to a point in his therapy where he began to contact some of these needs. In one session, he directly asked his therapist for some advice about how to handle a conflict with a friend; this was something he had never done before. The therapist responded by giving him advice and then asked him how it felt. He responded by tearing up, as he contacted the relief and gratitude toward the therapist for being willing to act on his behalf in this context and the underlying yearning for nurturance that had motivated his question.

In situations where therapists are unable to or choose not to gratify the underlying wish, it is important for them to be empathic and understanding while at the same time making it clear what their limits or boundaries are. It may, for example, be important for a patient to acknowledge her desire for the therapist to magically transform her and for the therapist to empathize with this desire, rather than to invalidate it. Or a therapist may not grant a patient's request to extend the session time, but nevertheless empathize with the desire. Or a therapist may empathize with the desire for personal contact between sessions without accommodating it and without denigrating it as merely transferential. In such cases, it is important to empathize with the underlying yearning and the pain and frustration that inevitably result from having the wish go unfulfilled. Through this process, patients gradually come to experience their therapists as being there for them.

Clinical Illustration

Often confrontation ruptures resolve over the course of a number of sessions, as the therapist and patient gradually and repeatedly work through earlier stages of the resolution process, thereby building the trust necessary to work through later stages. However, in some cases this process can take months or even years. In the following series of transcript excerpts, we illustrate the rupture resolution process as it unfolds over the course of a number of sessions for the patient identified as Joan in Chapter 4.

First Episode

CONFRONTATION MARKER

JOAN (J): Last week you asked me my understanding of how therapy works. And you didn't say very much in return. And now it's my turn. I want to know how the therapy you do works and how it's going to help me with my problems.

DISEMBEDDING

THERAPIST (T): I feel on the spot.

J: You had your chance last week. This week is mine. We're not wasting time this week!

T: Well, I'll try to give you a brief answer to your question. Basically, the way in which I work involves working with you to help you become aware of self-defeating patterns in your relationships with other people. Usually, this involves exploring your feelings and thoughts in problem situations, and often a fair amount of time is spent exploring things that go on in our relationship as a way of shedding light on things that may go on for you in relationships with other people.

J: But how is that going to help me?

T: Well . . . it's difficult to answer that in the abstract.

J: I'm not interested in an abstract answer. I want a direct, concrete answer.

T: I'd like to answer your question, but my experience is that I feel so pressured that it's difficult for me to think clearly.

J: Well, then say something that shows me how we're going to work so I can see what's going on.

T: See . . . even as you say that . . . I feel the same sort of pressure to perform.

J: Well, then say something meaningful.

T: I'd like to, but it feels to me like I'm trying and nothing I say satisfies you, so I feel at a loss.

J: Well, I don't want to give up.

Rather than responding directly to the content of Joan's question, the therapist metacommunicates his feeling of being "on the spot." This serves a couple of functions. First, the process of acknowledging an uncomfortable feeling helps to reopen internal space and free the therapist up to observe more clearly what may be going on in the interaction, rather than responding unconsciously out of his feeling of pressure. Second, it begins to ferret out the relational implications of Joan's question, as evidenced by her response, "You had your chance last week. This week is mine. We're not wasting time this week!" This suggests that Joan's question is not so much a genuine one coming from a place of openness and curiosity, but rather an angry demand for proof that the therapist can help her. Nevertheless, the therapist takes her question at face value since he may be wrong in his suspicion that no answer will be satisfactory for her. Moreover, to not answer the manifest content of the question may be experienced by the patient as disrespectful. Joan's responses ("But how is that going to help me?" and "Well, then say something meaningful"), however, deepen the therapist's sense that nothing he can say will satisfy her. Disclosing his experience of being stuck leads to a shift. Joan backs off and begins to express her fear of not being helped. Perhaps, too, there is an element of accommodation or compliance to her backing off.

EXPLORATION OF CONSTRUAL

T: It seems to me we have a shared dilemma here. My sense is that we're both trying as hard as we can, but that somehow we're stuck.

J: Well, don't you feel that last week was wasted?

T: I'm pretty clear about the fact that you're not happy with last week, and that's what counts.

J: Yeah . . .

T: Are you willing to tell me more about how it was wasted?

J: Nothing ever works. When I back off, like I did last week, it doesn't work, and when I hit people on the head, it doesn't work.

T: Okay . . . which are you doing right now?

J: Well . . . I guess I'm backing off a little.

T: What's that like for you?

J: Well . . . I guess I start to feel compromised. It's like I have to allow myself to be brainwashed in order to be helped.

T: That doesn't sound very good.

J: No.

T: Okay . . . so at the risk of oversimplifying, it sounds like you've got two basic strategies for getting what you want from people and that neither are really working. One is to kind of allow yourself to be brainwashed, to compromise yourself and somehow have something very important taken away from you. The other is to come out like a bull . . .

J: Both guns blazing. (*Chuckles.*)

T: Both guns blazing.

J: The first strategy is worse, because I end up chewing myself up and I feel worse.

T: So coming out with both guns blazing is the lesser of the two evils?

J: Yeah.

T: Okay . . . I don't know what the alternative is to these two strategies is for you, but I'm willing to work with you to find one. Does that sound worthwhile to you?

J: Yeah.

The therapist begins this segment by framing the situation in mutual terms in order to facilitate the development of the alliance ("we have a shared dilemma here"). In response to his probes, Joan is able to articulate her dilemma of having to choose between two unworkable strategies in order to get help: either compromising herself and allowing herself to feel brainwashed or being aggressive. Although it is only a beginning, we begin to get a glimpse here of the patient's relational schema. By probing Joan's experience in the moment, the therapist clarifies that even this momentary shift out of her aggressive stance is experienced by her as a compromise, but by empathizing with her dilemma ("That doesn't sound very good"), he may be able to reduce the obsta-

cle that this schema potentially presents to the sense of collaboration that is beginning to develop. He then attempts to facilitate the development of an alliance by suggesting a therapeutic goal that will make sense to Joan in this context: working together to discover an alternative to her current strategies of either compromising herself or approaching the other person with "both guns blazing."

One Week Later

J: I didn't get a chance to do what I figured out I'm gonna do, because I was too busy.

T: I'm unclear.

J: Well, my different tactics. Remember . . . one tactic didn't work, the second didn't work, so try a third one!

T: I see, so you're saying that you haven't come up with another strategy over the week.

Confrontation Marker

J: Oh yes I have! I just didn't get a chance to do it because it was a busy week, but I'll definitely have it in place by the next time (*grinning*).

T: I'm aware of your smile right now. Are you aware of it at all?

J: Yeah.

T: Yeah? What's your experience behind the smile?

J: I'm telling you where it's at and putting you down at the same time. I'm letting you know that you're not going to get the better of me.

This session begins with a confrontation marker mixed with features of a withdrawal marker. The therapist facilitates a more direct expression of her aggression by drawing Joan's attention to an interpersonal marker–her incongruent smile–and explores her experience. In response, she expresses her aggressive and self-protective sentiments in a more direct fashion: "I'm telling you where it's at and putting you down at the same time. I'm letting you know that you're not going to get the better of me."

DISEMBEDDING

T: Uhum . . . is this . . .

J: The same way that there's no reason for you not to have that water fountain fixed. [Joan is referring to a water fountain in the hallway which had been broken for some time. She had asked the therapist in passing at the beginning of the session if he was aware that it was broken, and he had casually responded that he did and that it had been broken for some time.] You knew it didn't work and you've done nothing about it. You didn't say you've tried to have it fixed and reported it. You're just like everybody else. I'm sick and tired of people treating me like dirt!

T: Wait a second. I'm feeling lumped in with everybody else right now.

J: Well, why not? You're a person. You're part of humanity. Why shouldn't you be lumped in with everybody else?

T: But I don't feel like I'm being treated like a person. It feels like you're lumping me in with everybody else.

J: Well, look at you! You're just like everybody else. You've known that thing doesn't work for ages, and what the hell did you do about it? The same thing that everybody else did. You deserve to be lumped in with everybody else. Do something that doesn't deserve being lumped in with everybody else!

T: I'm feeling reluctant to open my mouth.

J: Yeah ... well ... you just got one of my tirades (*looking sheepish*).

In response to Joan's tirade, the therapist discloses his experience of being "lumped in with everybody else." There is something impersonal about her attack, as though the therapist is simply another exemplar of the perpetrating object, rather than a specific individual whom she is angry at for his or her own actions. His comments, however, rather than helping them to disembed from the interaction, further infuriate her. When, however, the therapist comments on his "reluctance to open his mouth," for fear of triggering another tirade, something shifts.

AVOIDANCE OF AGGRESSION

T: What's happening for you now?

J: I'm feeling nervous.

T: What's your nervousness about?

J: Well, I told you my inner self, type of deal, and I know people don't like to have barrages like that. But then again, I don't really care, cause they deserve it.

T: Do you feel I deserve a barrage right now?

J: I'm careful when I do it, and only to people with whom I can get away with it.

T: But you're not answering my question.

J: I never answer questions (*laughing*). I always sidestep them.

T: Do you have an objection to answering this one?

J: Because what I really feel is unacceptable to people.

T: If possible, I'd like to personalize this. Do you feel that what you feel would be unacceptable of me?

J: Yeah. I'm pissed off at the world, and I have my fantasies of what I'd like to do to people.

T: What would you like to do to me?

J: I don't know. It's not the specific people in the world. Well, of course, if I could do what I wanted to do with you, I'd hit you in the head and make you present things to me the way I want you to (*looking away as she says this*).

T: Are you willing to actually make contact with me as you say this?

J: (*Chuckling*) Instead of looking away, where it's safe and impersonal?

T: Do you have any sense of what you're avoiding in not looking at me?

J: I guess it's kind of difficult for me to express my anger at you and tell you what I want, if I relate to you as a person. It's easier for me to think of you as an entity—as one of the masses of humanity that are out there.

T: Can you say more about your difficulty in relating to me as a person right now?

J: I don't know, but it has something to do with knowing that you're just like everybody else. I can't depend on anybody.

In response to the therapist's last effort to metacommunicate, Joan becomes self-conscious and anxious about the impact of her attack on him. The therapist attempts to explore the nature of her avoidance, and she responds in a generalized fashion (e.g., "people don't like to have barrages like that" and "what I really feel is unacceptable to people"). The therapist attempts to keep the exploration grounded in the here-and-now of the interaction in order to reduce the possibility of intellectualization and promote experiential discovery (e.g., "Do you feel that what you feel would be unacceptable to me?"). In response to Joan's global insinuation about her rageful fantasies about the world, the therapist again redirects her to the here-and-now of the therapeutic relationship ("What would you like to do to me?").

When Joan turns away, as she angrily expresses her desire for him to present things the way she wants, the therapist draws attention to her withdrawal and explores her avoidance. This is an illustration of the type of rapid shift in self-states described earlier. In response, Joan is able to begin articulating the nature of her avoidance more fully. Her statement that it is easier to relate to him as "one of the masses of humanity" than as a person supports the therapist's initial intuitions about "being lumped in with everybody else." She also hints at the underlying fear of abandonment that makes it difficult for the patient to be more vulnerable with the therapist.

Two Months Later

Joan arrives 10 minutes late for the session and begins without saying anything about being late.

RUPTURE MARKER (Confrontation Mixed with Features of Withdrawal)

J: I copied down what it says in the book last week, but it fell out of my purse, and I can't find it.

T: How do you mean you copied down what's in the book?

J: I told you about the book before. [The patient is referring to a book she has referred to previously which provides a popular account of a successful psychotherapy, although the therapist has not yet grasped this.] What's in the book?

DISEMBEDDING

T: I experience you as being kind of cryptic right now.

J: You're always asking me stupid questions. I mean exactly what I say. What's in the book?

T: I'll tell you what I'm guessing, okay? I'm guessing that you're . . .

J: I said I copied down what was in the book. It's a book about psychotherapy.

T: I'll tell you what's going on for me. I experience you as hinting at something, and I have . . .

J: What's difficult? What does "book" mean? What does "psychotherapy" mean? What does "copy" mean? I don't understand what's so difficult to understand. I don't use six-dollar words. I don't know them. If I did know them, I couldn't pronounce them, and I definitely couldn't spell them. So why do people find it difficult to understand me? I mean exactly what I said! And when I explain myself, people tell me that I ramble and get bored and don't listen to me. And when I cut out unnecessary words, they don't understand what I say. So what's a book? What does it say in the book?

Joan begins the session in a cryptic fashion. The therapist, while assuming that she is hinting at something negative, is genuinely puzzled, and attempts to clarify. Joan continues to be cryptic, and her comments begin to take on a condescending tone ("What's in the book?"). In an attempt to metacommunicate, the therapist reflects the cryptic quality of her communication, but says nothing about her condescending angry tone or his own affective response to it. Perhaps he is feeling too overwhelmed and anxious about his own internal response to comment on it? In response, Joan intensifies her attack.

DISEMBEDDING

T: I don't like the feeling of being treated like this.

J: Well, then don't treat me like that! And don't ask me what I mean. How could you not understand what I meant! I'm trying to find out what it is you don't understand. The word "book" or the word "copy"? What is it you don't understand?

T: I experience you as being very condescending toward me right now, and I don't like it.

J: I don't like you being condescending to me either. And what did you mean by "I don't understand you?"

T: I'm hesitating to say anything right now, because I'm . . .

J: What's there to hesitate about? Why can't you explain what you meant by "You don't understand," unless it was just a game you were playing?

T: See . . . my sense is that anything I might say will provoke you again, so I'm hesitating. (*Silence for approximately 1 minute.*) During this silence I think of things to say, but I feel cautious and concerned that anything I might say will strike you the wrong way.

J: What's the difference, anyways? I'm always getting told not to talk down to people and not to treat them like idiots. And when I try to treat them as if they know what's going on, they tell me I'm playing games.

The therapist finally addresses the hostile aspect of Joan's communication and his own response to it ("I don't like the feeling of being treated like this" and "I experience you as being very condescending toward me right now, and I don't like it"). By beginning to explicitly acknowledge some of his own negative feelings, by asserting himself, and by commenting on Joan's hostility, he begins to reestablish internal space for himself, within which he can process his experience more fully and be more present in the interaction with the patient. This can be understood as an "act of freedom" in Symington's (1983) sense. In addition, by beginning to convey some of his negative feelings to Joan in a modulated form, he begins to reestablish himself as a subject for her, rather than an object. Moreover, the ability to express his own negative feelings to her in a modulated form plays a role in ultimately helping to detoxify Joan's own negative feelings. Joan's immediate response is one of counterblame ("I don't like you being condescending to me either") and continued provocation ("And what did you mean by 'I don't understand you?' "). The therapist, sensing that any direct response will maintain or escalate the current cycle, metacommunicates his dilemma ("my sense is that anything I might say will provoke you again, so I'm hesitating").

Next he breaks the silent period that ensues, by metacommunicating his dilemma ("During this silence I think of things to say, but I feel cautious and concerned that anything I might say will strike you the wrong way"). This functions to prevent the silence from turning into a power struggle over who will break the silence and to reassure Joan that he is not completely abandoning her. Her response ("What's the difference anyways?") suggests that she may experience his comment as an attempt at reassurance, and her tone begins to shift from anger to hopelessness.

EXPLORATION OF CONSTRUAL

T: It feels like nothing you do works, huh?

J: As far as I'm concerned it's not a feeling. It's a fact.

T: Damned if you do and damned if you don't.

J: That's right. So what difference does it make?

T: So you just feel like giving up?

J: Well, sure. I've banged my head against a wall all my life. I read in the paper yesterday about a clairvoyant who predicted all kinds of disasters in the past, and now he's predicting another downswing in the economy and all kinds of global disasters. And you know, I think he's right.

T: What kind of predictions are you making for yourself?

J: I'm not even gonna bother. It's gonna be the same old garbage (*voice very low*).

T: Feeling kind of hopeless, eh?

J: I guess.

T: And I take it you're feeling pretty hopeless about things between us?

J: Oh yeah. I gave that up last week. After that breakthrough you managed to do 2 weeks ago, and then you threw it all away. Sure, that's why I didn't bother to make an effort to be on time today.

T: So you felt hopeless coming here today?

J: Well, I was defiant. What difference does it make whether I'm on time? Ten minutes here more or less doesn't make a damn bit of difference.

T: Uh-huh. So you're feeling hopeless and defiant?

J: Yeah.

The exploration of the Joan's feelings of hopelessness about the current interaction leads into a more general feeling of hopelessness about the future. As she begins to contact her feelings of hopelessness, Joan begins to externalize the feelings in terms of an article she read in a paper. The therapist redirects her to an internal focus and then to a focus on the therapeutic relationship. In response, she begins to talk about her feelings of disappointment over not feeling that they are maintaining the progress they made two sessions ago and then spontaneously acknowledges that her coming late to the session was a reflection of her hopelessness and defiance.

One Month Later

In the first part of the session, a characteristic theme for Joan emerges: her experience of being in a "can't win" situation with the therapist (i.e., if she expresses her anger directly, the therapist does not respond in a way that feels helpful to her, and if she attempts to hide her anger and go along with the therapist, she feels compromised and resentful). In the course of exploring this dilemma again, the patient becomes impatient and remarks:

CONFRONTATION MARKER

J: We've been through this before, and it's not getting us anywhere.

EXPLORATION OF CONSTRUAL

T: Uh-huh, so it's feeling futile.

J: Yeah. I can't afford to go on like this, doing nothing.

T: I hear a real sense of desperation in what you're saying.

J: Yeah, I guess so. I've been off work for a year and a half, and people are starting to wonder what the hell is wrong with me. And we've had some important sessions, but I still don't feel things changing.

T: Are you willing to tell me more about your feeling of desperation?

AVOIDANCE OF VULNERABILITY

J: I don't know. I try not to think about it.

T: What might happen if you were to explore it more deeply with me right now?

J: I think I'd start to feel even more hopeless, and then I'd be weak and pathetic.

T: Uh-huh. So there's something very uncomfortable about going into your feeling of hopelessness with me?

J: Yeah, I'm not sure I trust you to be here for me (*voice begins to crack*).

VULNERABILITY

T: What are you experiencing?

J: I feel sad.

T: Can you say anymore about your sadness?

J: I feel hurt and alone, and I don't know where to turn (*begins to sob*).

This segment begins with a habitual impasse for Joan and the therapist, and then proceeds to an exploration of Joan's construal of the futility of the situation. Because the way has been paved in previous sessions, no extensive process of disembedding from an enactment is required, and the exploration moves fairly quickly to her underlying feelings of desperation. As Joan touches on her feelings of desperation, she initially balks at the prospect of exploring them more fully. In response to the therapist's probing, however, she begins to contact her fears of abandonment, and this facilitates her ability to access underlying feelings of vulnerability and the need for nurturance.

✖ 6

Brief Relational Therapy

Over the last 15 years, we have been developing an approach to short-term treatment, based on the principles spelled out in this manual and consistent with many of the central features of the relational tradition. We call our model Brief Relational Therapy (hereafter referred to as BRT). The key characteristics of BRT are as follows:

1. It assumes a two-person psychology and a constructivist epistemology (or to be more precise, what Hoffman, 1998, refers to as a "dialectical constructivist" perspective).
2. It involves an intensive focus on the here-and-now of the therapeutic relationship.
3. It features an ongoing collaborative exploration of both patients' and therapists' contributions to the interaction.
4. It emphasizes in-depth exploration of the nuances of patients' experience in the context of unfolding therapeutic enactments and is cautious about making transference interpretations that speculate about generalized relational patterns.
5. It makes intensive use of therapeutic metacommunication and countertransference disclosure.
6. It emphasizes the subjectivity of the therapist's perceptions.
7. It assumes that the relational meaning of interventions is critical (see Aron, 1996; Mitchell, 1988).

Our primary impetus for developing BRT has been our interest in consolidating, refining, and empirically testing principles relevant to

resolving ruptures in the therapeutic alliance and potentially pernicious transference–countertransference enactments (e.g., Safran &
Muran, 1994, 1996; see Chapter 5). First at the Clarke Institute of Psychiatry in Toronto and subsequently at Beth Israel Medical Center in
New York City, we have been conducting research to evaluate the effectiveness of the treatment and to investigate the process through which
change takes place. This investigation of the mechanisms of change, in
turn, has helped us to refine the treatment model. At this point, we
have evidence that BRT is an effective form of psychotherapy for patients presenting with multiple psychiatric diagnoses, primarily in the
areas of depression and anxiety, with concomitant personality disorders. We also have preliminary evidence that BRT is more effective
than two more traditional approaches (a cognitive-behavioral and an
ego-psychological model) for patients with whom therapists find it
more difficult to establish a therapeutic alliance. These findings provide preliminary empirical support that the principles spelt out in this
book and implemented in the form of BRT are particularly useful for
negotiating problems in the therapeutic alliance and working through
treatment impasses.

Brief psychotherapy traces its origins to Sandor Ferenczi and Otto
Rank's (1925) pioneering attempts to counter the trend toward longer
analyses that was emerging at the time. It also reflected their interest in
emphasizing the experiential and relational aspects of treatment. Over
the years, a number of different models of brief psychodynamic therapy have been developed (e.g., Balint, Ornstein, & Balint, 1972; Malan,
1963; Mann, 1973; Sifneos, 1972). By and large, however, these developments have been regarded as "outside the pale" of mainstream psychoanalysis; indeed, in some respects they were devalued in the same
way that the supportive aspects of treatment were viewed as inferior to
the "pure gold" of psychoanalysis during the heyday of classical theory.
Currently, however, the psychoanalytic scene is undergoing tremendous ferment, and long-cherished theoretical and technical assumptions are being questioned (see Aron, 1996; Hoffman, 1998; Mitchell,
1997). At the same time, there are powerful economic and societal
pressures at play that make it advisable to ask serious questions about
what short-term approaches can and cannot offer, as well as what their
role should be within contemporary relational thinking.

In their authoritative book on brief psychodynamic therapy, Stanley Messer and Seth Warren (1995) categorize existing approaches
within Greenberg and Mitchell's (1983) distinction between drive/
structural and relational approaches. According to them, the drive/
structural approaches include those of Habib Davanloo (1980), David
Malan (1963), and Peter Sifneos (1972). These approaches all subscribe

to variants of an ego-psychological perspective and emphasize the interpretation of wish/defense conflicts as a central ingredient of change.
They tend to be quite confrontational in nature and by and large assume a one-person psychological perspective, paying little attention to
the therapist's contribution to enactments that take place. Messer and
Warren (1995) categorize the approaches of Lester Luborsky (1984),
Mardi Horowitz (1991), Joseph Weiss et al. (1986), and Hans Strupp
and Jeffrey Binder (1984) as relational approaches. They reason that
these four approaches can be characterized as relational because they
all conceptualize psychopathology in terms of recurrent maladaptive
patterns of interpersonal behavior. In these models, problems are conceptualized as arising from disturbances in relationships with early
caretakers that result in internal object relations, which pattern subsequent interpersonal relationships.

Although there is no doubt that on a continuum these four approaches are more consistent with a relational perspective than those
designated by Messer and Warren (1995) as drive/structural, in certain
respects they all fall short of a full-fledged relational model. It is beyond the scope of this chapter to provide a comprehensive critique of
these approaches from a relational perspective. In brief, however, we
can note that none of them are entirely faithful to the implications of a
two-person psychological perspective or of a constructivist epistemology, and none of them make the type of extensive use of the therapist's
countertransference as a source of information (and a potential focus
of self-disclosure) that is characteristic of relational approaches. Strupp
and Binder (1984), to a greater extent than the others do, emphasize
the notion that the therapist is a participant-observer and that his or
her feelings provide an important source of information. Even in their
approach, however, the tendency is to view the therapist as someone
who can step outside of the interpersonal field in order to develop a
more-or-less accurate formulation of the patient's core themes. This
type of stance contrasts sharply with the more radical view of contemporary interpersonal and relational theorists who argue that the therapist is always unwittingly participating in an enactment that he or she
can at best understand only partially (Aron, 1996; Levenson, 1983;
Mitchell, 1988; Renik, 1996; Stern, 1997).

THE DYNAMIC FOCUS

All the approaches described above call for the formulation of a dynamic focus early on in treatment (typically within the first three sessions). This emphasis on developing a case formulation early in the

process is viewed as critical given the brevity of the treatment. The understanding is that a focus of this type makes it possible to shorten treatment length by providing the therapist with a heuristic theory for guiding intervention in a systematic fashion. The focus thus becomes a thread that links apparently unrelated experiences together for both the therapist and the patient and allows the patient to gain some insight into and mastery over a central underlying theme in a brief period of time. It is the establishment of a dynamic focus and the consistent interpretation of that focus over time, as it emerges in a variety of different contexts, that facilitates the working through process and allows the patient to integrate treatment changes into his or her everyday life.

Although short-term therapists recognize that any dynamic focus is provisional and subject to revision, there is an inherent tension between the practice of using such a focus to guide one's interventions and certain tenets of a more constructivist/relational perspective. The formulation of a dynamic focus within the first few sessions of treatment is premised on the assumption that the therapist can stand sufficiently outside of the interaction to come up with an assessment of the patient's characteristic theme that is not shaped by the therapist's own unwitting participation in the interaction. From the perspective of a two-person psychology, this is impossible.

To be more fully consistent with the implications of a two-person psychological perspective, it is important for any case formulation that is developed to emerge gradually over time through the process of disembedding from whatever matrix is being enacted between therapist and patient. In this process, the therapist's understanding of the patient emerges only through his or her awareness of the nature of his or her own participation in the enactment, and this awareness always follows enactment (Aron, 1996; Levenson, 1983; Mitchell, 1997; Renik, 1996). Therapy thus consists of an ongoing cycle of enacting, disembedding, and understanding—and this understanding is always partial at best.

AWARENESS AND THE FOCUS
ON THE PRESENT MOMENT

This understanding of the therapeutic process is an important part of the guiding philosophy behind BRT. We have had to struggle with the problem of how to reconcile this principle with the time constraints of a brief-term treatment. This issue has two dimensions. The first concerns the question of how to maximize the probability that patients will be able to take something home with them, given the fact that there is no clear tangible focus that they can use to organize their experience and help them to gain a sense of mastery over their dilemmas. The second concerns therapists' anxieties about needing to offer something substantial to patients within a limited amount of time.

In terms of the first dimension, we replace the *content* focus of a dynamic formulation with a *process* focus on moment-to-moment awareness, or mindfulness. Of course, variants of characteristic themes do repeatedly emerge for patients, and the process of mutually acknowledging their importance helps to build the alliance. The point, however, is that we try to emphasize the process of discovery itself, rather than provide patients with any type of explicit formulation early in treatment. Moreover, we place less emphasis than many proponents of other short-term approaches do on the importance of repeatedly interpreting the same theme over the course of treatment.

Because this ambiguity can be anxiety-provoking for some patients, we attempt to foster the forging of the therapeutic alliance at the outset by providing patients with a clear rationale that emphasizes the importance of developing the capacity to observe their internal processes and their actions in relationship with other people as they are taking place. This capacity can be thought of as a type of mindfulness that is similar in many respects to what Peter Fonagy and Mary Target (1998) refer to as the ability to mentalize. Our emphasis on actively enlisting patients' collaboration in the task of self-observation resembles Gray's (1994) close process monitoring approach in some respects, but with an important difference. While Gray primarily emphasizes the task of intrapsychic self-observation, we also emphasize the importance of learning to observe one's own actions in interaction with others. At the outset of treatment we explain to patients that the therapeutic relationship is an important crucible for developing these capacities. Furthermore, we make it clear to our patients that therapy involves a process in which both patients and therapists work together to explore what is being unwittingly enacted in the therapeutic relationship and actively enlist their help in this process of collaborative exploration.

We wish to stress that *the emphasis in BRT is on developing a generalizable skill of mindfulness, rather than on gaining insight into and mastering a particular core theme.* This provides patients with a sense of something tangible that they can take away from the treatment, even if it is more abstract and nebulous than a sense of mastery over a particular theme. This is critical for purposes of facilitating agreement on both the task and the goal dimensions of the therapeutic alliance.

Our emphasis on the development of mindfulness also helps us to negotiate a thorny conceptual issue. If one takes the implications of a two-person psychology seriously, one is left with no guarantee that enactments taking place in therapy will parallel other relationships in the patient's life. Moreover, to the extent that there is a parallel, it will be partial at best. Thus, rather than emphasizing extratransference links, we encourage patients to monitor the extent to which relational patterns (both intrapsychic and interpersonal) that they have discovered through the exploration of therapeutic enactments take place in other relationships, and to refine their understanding of the nuances of their own relational patterns and associated internal processes through this type of ongoing awareness. This constitutes an important form of working through.

In addition, patients often spontaneously make links to other relationships when an emotionally immediate discovery takes place in the context of the relationship with the therapist. This, by the way, does not mean that we never make links to the patient's current life or genetic interpretations. We do so gingerly, however, and attempt to anticipate the relational meaning of the act to the patient. It is also important to explore our own motivations (e.g., is it a way of taking the heat off the therapeutic relationship or subtly blaming the patient?).

With regard to the second dimension (i.e., therapists' anxieties about the lack of a concrete focus), we strive towards Bion's (1967) ideal of approaching every session "without memory and desire." This entails an attempt to be aware of one's own preconceptions, as well as one's desire for things to be a certain way, and hence an acceptance of things as they are, a presentness and mutuality. We thus encourage the therapists we train to approach their work with the type of *beginner's mind* described earlier. To the extent that therapists can experience this state of mind, they increase their ability to relate to patients as subjects, rather than as objects (Buber, 1923).

This prescription is, of course, in many respects an unattainable ideal. Therapists inevitably have implicit formulations that influence their interventions. Thus the task is to try to become aware of these formulations, to use them to the extent they are helpful, and to move beyond them to the extent that they are not. Striving to approach things with a *beginner's mind* provides a useful corrective to the sense of purposeful striving that naturally emerges for therapists and that tends to become intensified in short-term therapy. The task for the therapist in BRT is thus not to let the time limit narrow the range of possibilities, but rather to attempt to realize the world of potential that resides in each moment of interaction by investing in it fully. The time limit is not something that needs to be ignored in order to allow this type of investment in the moment. Instead, ongoing awareness of the time limit can serve to intensify this investment.

Therapists are also encouraged to help their patients develop this type of heightened awareness of the present moment. In the same way that patients in classical theory are understood to develop an observing ego through identification with the observing ego of the analyst (Sterba, 1934), patients in BRT develop a heightened awareness of the present moment through identification with the therapist's stance in this respect. Our hope is that, in the words of William Blake, the patient will become better able to "to see the world in a grain of sand . . . eternity in an hour."

TERMINATION AND OPTIMAL DISILLUSIONMENT

Termination is an ever-present reality that colors the experience of both patients and therapists at conscious and unconscious levels. As in other forms of short-term therapy, in BRT the therapist and patient set a time limit at the beginning of treatment (e.g., 30 sessions), and that time limit becomes a critical part of the therapeutic frame. All approaches to brief dynamic therapy emphasize the importance of helping patients to work through the meaning of termination. Our approach, however, most resembles Mann's (1973) approach in the degree of emphasis that we place on termination as one of the central issues in treatment. We agree with Mann that the process of dealing with separation-individuation and loss is a central and ongoing struggle in life, and that the time constraints of brief-term therapy bring this struggle into high relief. As described earlier, we find it useful to broaden this conceptualization somewhat to think of human existence as entailing an ongoing dialectical tension between the need for agency and the need for relatedness (Aron, 1996; Bakan, 1966; Blatt & Blass, 1992; Safran & Muran, 1996; Winnicott, 1965). This tension is highlighted whenever problems emerge in the therapeutic relationship, and it is brought into relief in particularly accentuated form in the context of termination. Termination can be thought of as *the ultimate rupture in the therapeutic alliance.* Thus the termination process can provide a valuable opportunity for patients to learn to negotiate conflicting needs for agency and relatedness in a constructive fashion without disowning either of the two needs.

Reminding patients of termination periodically throughout the treatment and exploring their feelings about it is central to BRT. The purpose of this reminder is not to goad them into changing more quickly. Instead, it functions to heighten issues that are already there in latent form, thereby bringing to the surface conflicts and transference–countertransference dynamics that would often take considerably longer to emerge in long-term treatment. In response to reminders about the time limit, patients typically become more aware of and begin to explore whatever frustration, disappointment, and anger they have about not getting what they hoped they would get from therapy. The exploration of feelings about termination can lead in various directions. When patients begin treatment with a more aggressive or counterdependent stance, the therapist's work often involves surviving the aggression and ultimately working toward an exploration of the dependency and vulnerability that is being defended against (Winnicott, 1965). This typically resembles the resolution process for *confrontation ruptures,* described in Chapter 5. When patients begin treatment with a more dependent, deferential stance, the therapist's task is more likely to involve helping them to access angry feelings that are defended against, thereby giving them an opportunity to learn that the therapeutic relationship can survive their aggression (the resolution process for *withdrawal ruptures*). This, of course, is an oversimplification, since patients often present with features of both styles; nevertheless, it can be a useful heuristic.

A second common theme involves the exploration of the difficulties patients have in trusting and opening up to the therapist, given the time constraints. On the one hand, all relationships are transient, and we never know when an intimate relationship will disappear from our lives through death, a falling out, or some other circumstance beyond our control. Exploring patients' fears of abandonment in this context can open the door to an experientially real understanding of enduring attitudes (often unconscious in nature) that prevent them from opening up and finding intimacy in everyday situations. This type of exploration can help patients take the risk of investing in the relationship with the therapist despite its limitations (and despite the pain of loss that such an investment will inevitably entail).

At the same time, the legitimacy of patients' concerns about the time limit needs to be acknowledged by the therapist. In the same way that a therapeutic stance of abstinence and neutrality will have an inevitable impact on patients' experience, a predetermined time limit is more than just a symbolic reminder of the transience of all things. It is inevitably a form of abandonment. It is thus important for therapists to accept patients' reluctance to invest in the therapeutic relationship because of the time limit, as well as to validate and empathize with any pain and sadness that emerges through the exploration of feelings about termination. It is also critical for therapists to empathize with and validate feelings of anger that emerge in anticipation of abandonment by the therapist, as well as feelings of disappointment and resentment that patients experience around having not gotten all they hoped for from the treatment.

Dealing with patients' feelings about termination is often a critical turning point in the treatment. As we discussed earlier, it is common developmentally for people to learn to dissociate aspects of their basic needs or bodily-felt experience because of a failure of others to be optimally attuned to their needs (see Balint, 1968; Ferenczi, 1931; Winnicott, 1965). As a result, they learn to relate to others through a false self organization. As Winnicott (1965) in particular has emphasized, it is the therapist's failure that allows for the reenactment of the type of traumatic experience that is the by-product of the inevitable failure of patients' caretakers to be optimally responsive. And this in turn allows for a reworking of patients' relationships to the other and to their own needs in a new, constructive fashion. In BRT, the ongoing reminder of the time limit often heightens patients' awareness of their disappointment with the treatment and the therapist. Even though patients, at a conscious and rational level, may limit their expectations and hopes of what can be accomplished in 30 sessions of treatment, at an unconscious level they commonly harbor fantasies that the treatment will change their lives in a fundamental way. These fantasies will take different forms for different patients, but they all at some level reflect an idealized state of unity and perfection that in reality can never be attained.

If therapists can respond to their patients' disappointment or resentment as a legitimate response to limitations both of the treatment and of themselves, they can help them to access dissociated wishes and needs. The process of empathizing with these needs, even if they cannot be fulfilled, is critical because it helps patients to begin to accept them as valid and legitimate. At the same time, this process of acknowledging the limitations of the treatment and of one's own ability to be helpful, in tandem with empathizing with patients' disappointment, helps them to begin to accept the limitations of the other and to begin relinquishing their pursuit of an idealized and unattainable goal. In order for therapists to be able to tolerate patients' needs and disappointment in this context, they have to deal with their own fantasies of omnipotence and relinquish some of their own narcissistic strivings. This, of course, is true in any form of treatment, but conflicts of this type are heightened for therapists in brief-term therapy in the same way that they are for patients.

CASE ILLUSTRATION

In this section, we present a case in order to illustrate both BRT and the major principles we have outlined in this book.

The patient, Ruth, contracted to receive 30 sessions of BRT. She was an attractive, young-looking, 52-year-old woman, who had been divorced for 16 years and had a 22-year-old daughter. She worked as a high school teacher. She had ended her marriage of 12 years at the age of 36 because she felt her husband was controlling, emotionally abusive, and generally unable or unwilling to be responsive to her emotional needs. Since her divorce, she had had a series of short-term affairs with men that she herself typically ended because of her dissatisfaction with them. She had a tendency to get involved with people she looked down on and reported that she was afraid of pursuing men that she was more interested in for fear of being rejected. She maintained that in the past she had difficulty acknowledging to herself that she really wanted an enduring intimate relationship and that she had depended upon her physical attractiveness in order to seduce men into casual relationships, which were satisfying sexually and boosted her self-esteem. As she grew older, however, she became increasingly concerned that her appearance was deteriorating, that she would have difficulty continuing to attract men, and that she would possibly spend the rest of her life alone. At the beginning of treatment, she acknowledged that she desperately wanted to be in a "real relationship," but felt hopeless about the possibility. A second presenting problem revolved around her feelings of being "disempowered" and of not being treated respectfully by colleagues at work.

While the therapist initially felt very sympathetic toward her, a pattern developed fairly rapidly in which he had difficulty maintaining a sense of emotional engagement with her and found himself biding time until the sessions ended. Ruth had a tendency to tell long stories with considerable obsessional detail, and to do so in an unemotional droning fashion, which left the therapist feeling distant and unengaged. In addition, she rarely paused to welcome any input or feedback from the therapist, and this resulted in what seemed like an unending monologue, in which the therapist's presence was barely acknowledged. While he typically began sessions with a renewed intention of taking an interest in her, he consistently ended up feeling bored and vaguely irritated.

In an effort to understand what was being enacted between them, he began to metacommunicate about his emotional disengagement in an attempt to clarify potential links between his experience, her characteristic style of presentation, and the intrapsychic processes linked to it. She seemed quite responsive to his feedback, indicating that on various occasions she had received feedback of a similar kind from others in her life and that she was eager to try to understand how her own inner struggles and characteristic way of coping with them might be contributing to this dynamic. Over time, a mutual understanding of the cycle being enacted became fleshed out to some extent. She was able to articulate an underlying fear of abandonment that led her to defend against vulnerable feelings by controlling her style of presentation. She was also able to articulate a semiconscious perception of the therapist's disengagement and a tendency to intensify her deadening monologue as a way of dealing with feelings evoked by this perception.

Although on the one hand the therapist felt encouraged by her openness to exploring what was going on between them, he had an intuition that something did not feel quite right—perhaps an element of compliance in her response and a vague sense of himself beginning to play the sadistic role in a sadomasochistic enactment. At different points, he shared with her his sense that she seemed all too ready to work with whatever he presented. For example, he disclosed: "I have a complex reaction to your response. Let me see if I can put it into words. I make a comment like that, and there's a way in which you'll sort of take it and work very hard to make sense of it and look at yourself. On the one hand, I feel pleased that you're finding it useful . . . but on the other hand, I have a vague sense of discomfort . . . as if you're agreeing too readily . . . or I'm being coercive or something." At one level, the therapist felt that she seemed to take this in and work with it, but at another level he felt like even this response had an element of compliance.

The above notwithstanding, as the sessions progressed, the therapist did feel that a degree of trust was developing and that Ruth was beginning to open up. In retrospect, Session 15 turned out to be a particularly important one. Ruth came to the session feeling stuck and despondent and filled the hour with a litany of her somatic problems (sinus problems, headaches, etc.). During this session, the therapist struggled with his own sense of helplessness and impotence in the face of Ruth's inertia. However, by recalling his own feelings of helplessness in the face of various somatic problems he had experienced over the years, he was able to identify with Ruth. This helped him to accept his own feelings of impotence with her and to listen to her complaints in a reasonably accepting and empathic fashion, without giving into the urge to solve her problems or to push her to be some place other than where she was. As we will see, this subsequently turned out to be important for Ruth.

Ruth began the following session with a rather complex and difficult-to-follow story about a stray dog that she had found and decided to keep. Because she had felt that it would be too burdensome to look after her dog all by herself, she asked some neighbors to help her with it by keeping it at their place sometimes. The arrangement had worked reasonably well for a brief period, but now the neighbors were saying that it was emotionally harmful for the dog to go back and forth between houses, and they wanted exclusive possession of the dog.

After listening to an extended, uninterrupted monologue about the problem, the therapist finally interrupted and metacommunicated to her:

THERAPIST (T): I find myself poised to start talking with you about it . . . but sort of waiting for an opening.

RUTH (R): Oh . . . okay . . .

T: I also find myself wondering a little bit about the extent to which you're really wanting or inviting my input.

R: I really do.

T: You do?

R: Well . . . I want it to whatever extent you feel comfortable getting involved.

T: Yeah?

R: I mean . . . I guess . . . that's why there's a hesitancy . . . I guess there's an assumption on my part . . . that you don't want to be involved . . . that you're throwing it back to me.

T: So it sounds like you're reluctant to directly ask me for my help, because you assume I won't respond.

R: Yeah.

T: Do you have a sense of what would feel helpful . . . of what you would like from me?

R: Well . . . what should I do? Should I fight for the dog or let him go?

T: Before I answer . . . I wonder if you can say anything about what it feels like to say this?

R: Umm . . . (*voice shaky*) I think it's a really . . . it's really hard for me to say . . . what I want . . . and it's even harder . . . and why I think it's so hard is it's . . . I can't imagine that I'll get it. You know that, umm . . . and I've really just become aware of how . . . kind of at such a core level, there is this kind of . . . a sense of having been disappointed in getting what I want.

T: Uh-huh.

R: So, I mean, I think that's, you know, umm . . . kind of a very big defense I have, like kind of shrouding what I want in a way. I think there was something that happened last week, when I was talking about being depressed and not feeling well . . . where you seemed sympathetic and didn't minimize my anguish, either physically or psychologically . . . and I know that it had a very big effect on me. So I guess I feel much more trusting. In a way, it's funny because it's almost like a painful thing cause it's so umm . . . yeah . . . it's like, it just sort of opens up this door, you know?

As this segment suggests, the therapist's ability to provide a holding or containing function for Ruth during the previous session appears to have helped her to become more trusting and to have brought her desire for nurturance closer to the surface. Initially, her fear of abandonment gives rise to a characteristic interpersonal marker for her, that is, a rather circumstantial monologue. However, the therapist's metacommunication about her impact on him (i.e., his feeling of uncertainty about whether she wants his input) appears to help Ruth express her desire for help more directly.

Subsequent to a more extended exploration of Ruth's feelings about asking for and receiving help, the therapist did give his opinion about how to handle the dog situation. Ruth seemed to find his willingness to do so important. Despite the apparent importance of these last two sessions for Ruth, the next two sessions seemed relatively uneventful. But, an important shift took place in Session 19, which she began by telling the therapist about how she had experienced a minor comment of his at the end of the previous session as particularly validating. During this previous session, she had been talking about a situation at work in which she had been feeling chastised and infantilized by the school principal and had been feeling powerless to change the situation. Since they were coming to the end of the session, the therapist had remarked, "This seems like something important to talk about. There are some important issues here."

When he then asked Ruth what she had found helpful about his comment, she remarked that it had reassured her that he didn't think she was petty or that she was responsible herself for setting up the problem situation at work. At the same time, she began to wonder out loud about the fact that she had such a lack of confidence that his minor comment at the end of the session was so important to her. When the therapist responded that he had been wondering about the same thing, she spontaneously connected it to times in the past when he had metacommunicated about his feelings of being disengaged from her and she had responded by attempting to work with his observations. At this point, she began to shift the topic. The therapist encouraged her to explore what occurred internally in the moment prior to the shift. She responded: "What came to mind is 'Well, that's probably good because I'm a good patient,' and then I thought of saying, 'Well, now I want to be a bad patient. Like now I don't want to be nice.'" This led into a story about a friend of hers, who had been in therapy and had one day knocked her therapist's books off the shelf in anger. In the remainder of the session, they began to explore the way in which her tendency to comply was an attempt to be a "good girl," a theme that cut across many situations for her.

In the following session, Ruth began for the first time to complain more directly about what she felt she wasn't getting from the therapist in treatment. While the previous session had felt to the therapist like a preliminary playing with the possibility of acknowledging her dissatisfaction, in this session her frustration, anger, and disappointment were more tangible. She began the session by indicating that she was aware of the fact that the treatment was more than halfway through and by asking for an evaluation of how things were going so far and for a plan for the rest of the treatment.

R: How many sessions do we have left?

T: Ten more, including today.

R: Okay . . . okay . . . so ten more. Oh my God . . .

T: So what's the "Oh my God?"

R: Well . . . I certainly don't feel like everything's resolved . . . you know . . . and (*clears throat*) umm . . . how can we speed it up (*laughs*)? Well, you know, I don't know if just coming here and complaining and being teary . . . if that's really the most productive thing.

T: It sounds like you're feeling kind of frustrated. Can you say any more?

R: Well . . . I guess I feel like asking you for an evaluation . . . or how we should proceed or something.

T: I don't want to sound evasive . . . but I'm not sure how to answer your question at this moment. Maybe we'll be able to come back to it later, and I'll be able to answer it in a way that feels helpful. But I'm wondering how you're feeling about what's going on between us in this moment?

R: Well . . . I mean . . . I don't feel like I'm blaming you in any way. I just think that it's easy for me to get sidetracked . . . and I may need help being reined in a little. I just feel like I need to have some concrete . . . not direction . . . I don't know . . . I feel like I need help being brought back on topic. And as we've discussed, when I don't know what the other person is thinking I tend to go on and keep throwing lines out in an attempt to get a response.

T: So part of it is that you want me to help you keep focused. . . . And are you also saying that you'd feel more comfortable if I were more forthcoming about what's going on for me?

R: Well, I guess so. I mean sometimes I feel like there's some kind of real connection that goes on, and then other times I think I'm totally spinning this yarn, and you know . . . you're just waiting for me to come back or something.

T: It sounds like your sense of how connected we are . . . how engaged I am and how much I'm there for you . . . fluctuates.

R: Uh-huh. I mean . . . I don't think that you don't like me, but I think this has been hard work. And hard work for you too. And I know from working with people . . . you like them the best when they make you feel good about what you're doing. And I don't know if I've been a success story.

T: Uh-huh.

R: So you know . . . when somebody . . . when I'm feeling like embraced . . . you know . . . totally accepted . . . like purely and unconditionally . . . then I'm more relaxed in a way.

T: Right . . . and you haven't always gotten that sense from me.

R: Right. Yeah.

T: That at some fundamental level . . . that I'm here for you and feel good about you.

R: Right. There's a reservation. And I think I'm always trying to figure out where the other person is . . . like feeling their pulse in a way.

This session contains many of the features of the resolution process for withdrawal ruptures. Ruth begins by indicating her concern about the lack of time. When the therapist attempts to explore her feelings, she responds with a series of qualified assertions in which she simultaneously expresses her negative feelings and associated demands (e.g., "I certainly don't feel like everything's resolved . . . how can we speed it up?") and qualifies them or attempts to soften their impact ("I don't feel like I'm blaming you in any way"). Rather than directly blaming the therapist for the lack of progress, she has a characteristic style of openly blaming herself, while implicitly blaming the therapist and asking for more help. She conceptualizes the problem primarily as resulting from her own lack of focus, but implicitly blames the therapist for not helping her to be more focused. The therapist acknowledges her request for help with focusing, but highlights her concerns about his opaqueness. Whereas Ruth expresses her concerns in a diffuse or self-blaming fashion ("sometimes I feel like there's some kind of real connection that goes on, and then other times I think I'm totally spinning this yarn"), the therapist highlights his contribution ("It sounds like your sense of how connected we are . . . how engaged I am and how much I'm there for you . . . fluctuates"). This leads to the emergence of Ruth's deeper concerns about his not really caring about her.

T: So . . . how am I doing right now?

R: I think that you're receptive . . . but I also want to know about my perceptions so far. I want you to tell me if I'm right or not. Are my perceptions accurate or distorted?

T: Well . . . I think you're right that my feeling of engagement fluctuates. . . . We've talked about this before to some extent. But also, it feels to me that I've been feeling increasingly more engaged over the last few sessions.

R: And your feeling disengaged relates to my wandering and losing focus?

T: I'm not completely sure . . . but I think so . . .

R: Well, then in the time we have left I want you to help me stay focused. And I also want to know why I drift away. Okay? So where do we go from here?

T: I'm not sure . . . but I'm wondering if you can say anything about how my feedback felt for you . . . and also when you say, "Where do we go from here?," what you're feeling?

When the therapist answers in the affirmative to Ruth's direct question about whether his feelings of engagement with her fluctuate, she responds by once again suggesting that she wants help staying focused. She then continues to place the ball in his court by asking him, "Where do we go from here?" The therapist, sensing the angry feelings underlying her words, attempts to explore her reaction to his feedback.

R: It's like . . . I'm not going to take all the responsibility.

T: So . . . is there a sense maybe . . . that it feels like I've been blaming you?

R: Yeah . . . I guess so. It's like I've really sincerely tried to get to important things . . . and it's like . . . I guess I'm asking for your help.

T: Okay . . . so that sounds important . . .

R: Yeah . . .

T: It's like you're saying "I'm really doing everything I can."

R: Right. It's not like you have to keep prodding me to get me to say what I feel. You might in a certain way . . . but I think I've been very forthcoming about my feelings as far as I know them.

T: Right. And you're basically saying "I need help. I want more from you."

R: Right.

T: What does that feel like to say, "I want more from you"?

R: Well, I immediately want to qualify it. I mean . . . I need more from you because we only have 10 sessions . . . so we need to work faster.

In this segment of the transcript, the therapist facilitates self-assertion by empathizing with the feelings and wishes that are implicit in the things that Ruth is saying. Underlying Ruth's explicit requests that he help her focus and her attempts to put the ball in his court is a deeper desire for him to be there for her and help her in a more fundamental way. Ruth agrees with his interpretation or empathic articulation of her underlying wish. When he explores the feelings associated with acknowledging this wish, however, she begins to contact her avoidance.

T: So it sounds like it's uncomfortable to ask for what you want from me.

R: Yeah.

T: Can you say anything more about your discomfort?

R: Well . . . It's like I'm being unreasonable and expecting too much . . . but still . . . I have a tendency to blame myself when things aren't going well in a relationship. And I don't want to do that here.

T: Yeah. It's not really fair for you to have to take all the blame if things don't work out for you here . . .

R: If I'm not to blame. I'm asking you to be really honest and tell me if I go off and start talking about a crack in the ceiling or whatever. Actually, as I'm saying that, I'm feeling stronger.

T: Uh-huh . . . and the essence of what you're saying in feeling stronger . . . is that you want me to take some of the responsibility for what's going on . . . and you don't want to feel blamed for something that's not your fault . . .

R: Yeah . . . And I just had a thought, "I want this time to be about me."

T: Uh-huh.

R: I don't want this to be a kind of academic observation . . . and I'm demanding that you be engaged in whatever problems I have . . . as mundane as they may be, as repetitive as they may be.

T: That sounds important. What does it feel like to say that?

R: Well . . . I feel like I'm stamping my feet in a way. You know . . . like "Goddamn it!" (*Laughs.*) You know . . . like "Give me that!"

T: Right.

R: But you know . . . it feels okay to say it . . . and actually I don't know that I thought this consciously at all . . .

T: Uh-huh.

R: But I guess a momentum is building, and I'm becoming more self-centered in it, like I want this to be about me and it should be.

T: Right.

R: And then the defensive part of me thinks, "It has to be about me . . . the person that I am . . . I can't try to be a more interesting person for you to be more engaged."

T: I don't see how that's defensive. Basically, you're saying "I want to be accepted on my own terms . . . for who I am."

R: Yeah . . . yeah . . .

T: And that sounds important. You know . . . I think that part of what you're saying is that when I tell you that my attention is wandering, you're feeling, "The hell with you! I want you to accept me for who I am."

R: Yeah. Exactly.

The exploration of Ruth's avoidance helps her to articulate and recognize the self-criticism that blocks the direct expression of her underlying wish. This helps her to bypass the self-criticism and move once again toward expressing feelings and wishes that have been avoided. At first, she continues to frame things in terms of the therapist helping her to focus. Perhaps this presentation can be understood as a continued compromise between the underlying wish to be helped and her self-critical form of avoidance. In other words, the problem in her mind is still her lack of focus, but she wants the therapist's help with this problem. The therapist empathizes with the aspect of her communication that emphasizes her desire for him to take responsibility for what is going on in their relationship. This helps her to contact and assert her underlying wish for him to be engaged and to accept her for who she is. Her statement, "I don't want this to be a kind of academic observation," suggests that she has been experiencing the therapist as distant and detached, rather than as personally involved. Given the difficulties the therapist has had feeling emotionally engaged (although this has been shifting over time), this is not surprising.

In contrast to the previous session, there were times in this session when the therapist felt strongly chastised, pressured, and momentarily at a loss as to how to respond to her pressure. At the same time, Ruth's ability to express her need for more emotional engagement helped him to empathize more fully with the experience of not feeling accepted and validated by him. In this and subse-

quent sessions, she was also able to contact sad and painful feelings of being hurt by his failure to accept and prize her in the way she wished him to. This led to a subtle but irrevocable shift in his perception of her. During periods in which her characteristic droning style of speaking continued, he found himself more engaged than he had been in the past. It was as if he was now unable to experience this aspect of her without simultaneously seeing her as a whole person with hopes, dreams, and frustrated yearnings.

As discussed previously in Chapters 3 and 4, there will inevitably be both subtle and not-so-subtle levels at which we, as therapists, fail to accept our patients. Only by becoming aware of and acknowledging the ways in which we are not being fully accepting can we become more so. This process of becoming more accepting involves an active engagement in ongoing dialogue with the patient, in which the therapist judiciously shares aspects of his or her subjective experience in an attempt to facilitate an exploration of what is being enacted in the relationship. Thus, with Ruth, the process of metacommunicating about his difficulty staying engaged with her helped the therapist to make explicit that which was already implicit—that is, his difficulty being there for her in a present and attuned fashion on a consistent basis. By acknowledging to himself and to Ruth an aspect of his experience that made it difficult for him to be more accepting, a process was initiated that ultimately allowed him to become more present and emotionally available.

At the same time, however, the therapist's metacommunication about his difficulty staying engaged did not constitute a complete disembedding from the vicious cycle that was being enacted; instead, it was a new step in the dance that was already taking place. By encouraging Ruth to tell him about the impact of his metacommunication on her and by being receptive to her feedback, the therapist was able to develop a greater empathic appreciation of her dilemma, in part as a result of his increased experiential appreciation of the way in which he has become a perpetrator in the relationship. The experience of challenging the therapist and seeing that their relationship was able to survive this challenge enabled Ruth to subsequently bring her feelings of despair, as well as her vulnerability and dependency, more fully into the relationship.

Ruth began the following session by talking about the fact that although she had left the previous session "all fired up" and ready to make changes in her life, she found herself sinking back into an apathetic inertia. As she spoke about her experience of inertia and sense of hopelessness, she began to sound slightly tearful.

R: I'm struggling with the question "What can I do to stay on track?"

T: I'm also feeling that at least implicitly you're asking me for my help here. Does that fit?

R: Yeah . . .

T: I'm struggling with your question because I don't want you to feel abandoned here. But I'm also feeling a little stuck.

Despite Ruth's progress in the previous session toward asserting her wish for the therapist to accept her and be there for her, here she reverts back to an interpersonally disconnected sense of hopelessness and aimlessness. The therapist metacommunicates his intuition that Ruth's complaints and her description of her struggle are, at least in part, an implicit request for help. This helps Ruth to acknowledge her implicit plea for help. The therapist is then faced with a dilemma. He knows how difficult it is for Ruth to ask for help and is concerned that a failure to make an effort to be responsive to her request will leave her feeling abandoned and at fault about acknowledging her desire for help in the first place. At the same time, he is not immediately clear on how to respond in a fashion that will be experienced as helpful. He thus metacommunicates his dilemma to her.

R: So . . . (*begins to cry and then stops herself*).

T: What's happening?

R: Well, I guess . . . I guess it probably comes back to sort of . . . our kind of not being connected or not having this kind of umm . . . natural kind of rapport. In a way, I mean, I think you know that it's your job not to let me leave here feeling worse after 30 weeks or something and umm . . . Yeah, and I think you would feel like you failed. Umm . . .

T: A moment ago, there were some real tears and sadness, and I'm wondering if you have a sense of what was going on there. (*Pause.*) It seemed to have to do with when I said "I don't want you to feel abandoned."

R: Umm . . . (*pauses*). I guess if that's the reason, then I'm abandoned anyway (*crying*).

T: How so?

R: (*Pause.*) I guess it would be some superficial . . . artificial you know, wrapping up . . . umm . . . I just had the sense that it was kind of "Now we have to work on this closure" and I'm certainly not . . . there are a lot of loose ends. (*She struggles to control her crying for a period of about 10 seconds.*)

The therapist's metacommunication about his dilemma results in a deepening of the alliance rupture. Further exploration reveals that Ruth experiences his response as a confirmation that he does not really care for her in a personal way and that his desire to help is motivated by a sense of professional responsibility.

T: It's like you're really struggling internally right now.

R: (*Sobbing in a controlled fashion and looking downward*) Yeah, I guess, you know, I just think . . . that for whatever reason this situation has brought out so much of my sadness and loss and disappointment, and that instead of me feeling like I'm going forward, I just feel like I keep on uncovering things that I'm not even that aware of. I mean, I know they're there, but . . . I don't know.

T: So, a couple of things come to mind, but one is . . . you know . . . I'm very aware that in this moment you're looking down . . . looking away from me. Do you have a sense of that?

R: Well, yeah . . .

T: Yeah?

R: I mean I do . . . because I just . . . I want to push it back in, and it just feels so umm . . . I mean, I feel it's about nothing. It just seems like this endless self-pity or something and umm . . .

T: So, what would happen if you didn't push your experience back in there?

R: I couldn't deal . . . I just (*brief pause*) would be blubbering and not even able to talk. You know, it's so embarrassing. It's not like . . . I mean, I know I'm not looking, and it's almost like I want to go away from you . . . like be by myself in a way.

T: Well, so part of what's happening I think is that you're, in your pain and sadness right now, you're pulling away from me . . . you're isolating yourself from me.

R: Uh-huh.

T: That seems important to me.

R: Does that, does it feel like that, or is . . . ?

T: Yeah, it does feel like that.

R: It does?

T: Yeah, You're . . . you find it . . . you're finding it difficult to, in some way, let me be here for you and for you in your pain right now . . . and I have a sense of not being let in. (*Long pause.*)

In a simple fashion, the therapist metacommunicates his observation that Ruth is looking down as she is crying. This helps her begin to articulate the internal processes leading to the avoidance of her sadness. She condemns herself for her tears, viewing them as a form of self-pity. In terms of the rupture resolution model, this would be viewed as the exploration of a self-critical form of avoidance. Developmentally, this self-criticism can be understood as an intro-

ject or an internalization of the negative attitudes of significant others. Further exploration helps her begin to articulate the aspect of her avoidance that involves current expectations of others. She finds it embarrassing to cry in front of the therapist. At this point, rather than continuing to explore the internal aspect of her avoidance, the therapist draws her attention to the interpersonal function of what she is doing: she is withdrawing from him. In CCRT terms, this can be understood as a response of self, that is, she isolates herself because of her anticipation of abandonment. This is a critical point in the process. Ruth experiences the therapist as abandoning her without experiencing the way in which she isolates herself from him. The therapist's intervention, however, has been at an interpretive level, that is, he is speaking about his understanding of what she is doing, rather than his experience of it. Ruth then asks him to speak from his experience. Perhaps this is particularly critical for her because of her general sense that the therapist is relating to her in a somewhat distant professional fashion, rather than as one human being caring for another. At first, he seems to have difficulty responding at a personal level ("You're finding it difficult to let me be here for you"). He then, however, goes on to disclose his own "sense of not being let in."

R: I don't know if I do know how to share that or probably lots of other things. I don't know. I mean, as much as I want to not feel like I'm doing everything wrong, it's such an embarrassment almost to . . . to . . . to even feel like I'm, you know, letting someone feel like I'm depending on them. And part of it is because (*brief pause*) that almost forces you to be there, you know (*brief pause*) and that makes me uncomfortable, I guess. I mean, I think I'm so . . . like if somebody wants to be there, they have to want to be there.

T: Right . . .

R: Not because . . . I expect anything or am depending on them.

T: Yeah, and you're saying that part of your reluctance to share your pain with me is that you don't want me to feel pressured in a way.

R: Yeah, and having to give me something that you don't want to, or that, that you feel you must . . . you know.

The therapist's disclosure of feeling kept outside seems to trigger an important exploratory process. In an experientially grounded fashion, Ruth articulates her discomfort with depending on others and her fear that the other (in this case the therapist) will be there for her out of a sense of pressure or obligation, rather than because of spontaneous caring.

T: Well . . . do you have any sense of how I'm responding to whatever pain you're showing?

R: Well, I think you're working harder.

T: What's that like for you?

R: Umm . . . Well, I guess it's a little uncomfortable.

T: Can you say more?

R: Well . . . I mean . . . it's so unfamiliar in a way. You can imagine what you want . . . you know . . . but then experiencing it, even if it is what you want, isn't always easy.

T: What are you experiencing?

R: Well, I guess it's just how . . . (*pause with some crying*) how much I really do want to feel involved or, you know . . . close to someone . . . and how simultaneously it's really somehow painful. (*Pause.*)

T: Can you say any more about the pain you're feeling? The pain of . . .

R: (*Crying*) I don't know quite why, umm . . . (*pause for 15 seconds*). I think part of it is that, umm . . . you know, it's like when you're holding everything together, it's so kind of . . . oh God, what's the word, you know . . . just holding on so tight and really defended and then suddenly when you don't . . . it's a relief on one hand. But then the whole other side of it, you know, of being defended and holding it all in. It's like, umm . . . because it's been so squelched, then it just sort of spills out. So I think, I don't know what I think . . . I'm just . . . lost there. (*Pause for about 20 seconds.*) Though I do think it makes me feel . . . (*still crying a bit*) umm . . . kind of the loss of what's been missing, or what is missing, an absence of that, and . . . and that makes me sad.

T: Just stay with what you're feeling right now, if you can. What are you experiencing?

R: (*Deep sigh.*) Well . . . (*pause for 15 seconds and crying again*) . . . it's just that I feel I've spent so much time playing this sort of game that has nothing . . . it's so removed from this place. So that whatever I got . . . kind of never touched me in a way. I've spent a lot of time acting like I didn't care about things and didn't care about people or wasn't serious, and whatever I was getting then . . . you know . . . I still wasn't getting it because it wasn't about what I really needed. I was never putting that out there.

T: Right.

R: . . . and the loss of all of that time, it . . . it makes me sad.

T: So, in touching some of your sadness right now . . . and having some sense of my . . . at least trying to be here for you in your sadness . . .

brings up even more sadness, a sense of loss, like a sense of having gone for so long without this.

R: Yeah.

Since the therapist is feeling genuinely caring toward Ruth, there is the potential for a valuable new relational experience. Given Ruth's readiness to perceive the other as abandoning or as responding out of a sense of pressure, however, it seems important to explore her experience of the quality of his responsiveness. Her response suggests that she does experience (at least to some extent) the therapist as genuinely caring in the moment. This evokes her own feelings of discomfort with the degree of intimacy, and this in turn evokes a host of complex feelings and associations. What stands out as particularly important here is that Ruth appears to have an experientially powerful awareness of the way in which her own lack of acceptance of her wish for nurturance and caring has made it difficult for her to establish satisfying and intimate relationships. Her sadness and pain at the end can be understood at different levels. At one level, it can be understood as a natural response to the experience of loss associated with the recognition of the role that her self-defeating relational matrix has played in robbing her of caring. At another level, it can be understood as the emergence of painful, warded-off feelings in response to the therapist passing a transference test (Weiss et al., 1986).

In subsequent sessions, Ruth explored her fears and sadness about imminent abandonment by the therapist, as well as her anger. She began Session 23 by talking about her fears of abandonment in general.

R: I have this general fear of being abandoned and disappointed. And so I guess I just shut down and cut people out of my life.

T: In the back of my mind, I'm thinking that we only have six or seven more sessions, and so I'm wondering about this whole issue of opening up and being abandoned in this context.

R: Well, it does make me sort of scared when I start thinking about the ending. And I guess that's true of me in general. I guess I'm reluctant to really involve myself deeply in relationships, but the desire is still there.

T: Uh-huh ... I have a sense of a real yearning inside of you.

R: (*Begins to cry and then stops herself.*)

T: What's happening for you?

R: Well, it starts to hurt, and then I think, intellectually, it's so inappropriate for me to be upset about therapy ending.

T: It doesn't seem inappropriate to me. We've worked together for a while now and we've really started to develop a relationship, and my sense is that you're beginning to open up and trust. And we're ending soon, and that's got to be painful.

R: Well, and I guess part of it is the finiteness of it. I leave with whatever feelings I have, and for you, it's like "Good. That was a tough one. That's over." And then you go on with something else.

This last remark led to a discussion of the inequity of the situation and her anger at the therapist. She also spontaneously drew a parallel between her experience of his lack of equal investment in their relationship, and a general tendency for men she had felt deeply about to not reciprocate the depth of her feelings.

In the following session, the theme of inequity emerged once again. Ruth returned to her concern that the therapist would be glad when things are over, because he found her frustrating and difficult to work with. While it was true that the therapist had felt frustrated, bored, and disengaged from Ruth, especially in the earlier part of the treatment, he was now experiencing their sessions as vitally alive and engaging. He had a growing feeling of empathy for her dilemma, felt deeply moved by her pain, and very much understanding of her feelings of anger toward him. In his own mind, he struggled with the question of whether he should say anything to her about the change in his feelings toward her. He tentatively resolved not to say anything, trusting that she would be able to experience the change in his feelings at an affective level, and fearing that verbal reassurances would be experienced by her as hollow. She then spontaneously told him that she didn't want him to tell her whether she was right about his feelings, because if he denied it, she might not believe him, and if he didn't, she would be upset.

Further exploration helped her to flesh out her concerns about his feelings toward her and to articulate her desire for him to really care about her. The process of putting this into words led to more sadness, but also to a feeling of satisfaction about her ability to take the risk of saying this. The session ended with her returning to her feelings of hurt and anger about the fact that the therapist had not volunteered to meet beyond the preestablished termination session. He empathized with her feelings and told her that he believed it was legitimate for her to feel both hurt and angry with him.

She began Session 28 by talking about the fact that she normally had difficulty trusting that men are interested in her or care about her, unless they go overboard in their attempts to woo her. When they did do this, however, she reported finding that she loses herself in the process. She maintained that given this, she felt good about the fact that she was starting to feel okay about her relationship with the therapist, despite the fact that he had not actively reassured her. She told a story about a recent encounter with a male friend, in which she had difficulty trusting that he would be there for her, despite evidence to the contrary.

T: It sounds like normally there's a real lack of faith that relationships will work out.

R: Yeah (*appears touched by this*). That really captures something important. Normally, I tend to devalue relationships when I don't get much active reassurance from people. And I guess there's a risk of my doing that to some extent with our relationship, because you're not proposing that we extend our meetings.

T: What I'm thinking is that you really need and deserve somebody to be there for you on an ongoing basis, and I'm wondering if you can still find anything of value in our relationship, despite the fact that I'm not going to be there for you in the future in the way you deserve.

R: (*Beginning to cry slightly*) I'm thinking about it, and I think it's okay. I don't feel abandoned by you. I'm sad, I think, because I'm so aware in this moment of the way my lack of faith in people and fear of abandonment have acted as obstacles to my getting into a good relationship. And I'm thinking about my daughter as well . . . how her lack of faith in relationships gets in the way. I know this is a bit of a digression, but I guess I'm identifying with her . . . This is an important place to come to. And I thought I wasn't going to cry today (*said with a slightly humorous tone followed by a short period of silence*). I feel like thanking you, and then saying goodbye (*said quickly in a humorous tone*).

T: This feels like an awkward moment?

R: Yeah. It feels a little difficult staying with the feeling of contact with you.

T: So some of what's going on is that along with the pain you feel a sense of connection with me and of gratitude. That's what's uncomfortable?

R: Yeah. Any sort of closeness. It's almost like I have to cut that feeling. I think one time we talked about how I start to feel suffocated when I feel intimate.

T: Can you say any more about this feeling of suffocation?

R: I guess it's something about the welling up of all these emotions. There's some part of me that always wants to push it down. I don't know what would happen if I didn't. I don't know if it's about being exposed or being out of control. I don't know. But I want to contain it. It's bigger than the both of us (*laughing . . . then pause*). I don't know what love really is. I think I have it with my daughter, but even that . . . it's not direct. The direct expression of feelings is very hard.

T: Uh-huh. I was wondering when you said "It's bigger than the both of us." I know you were laughing, but it sounded interesting.

R: Well, when you ask what am I afraid of . . . I'm afraid that feelings . . . they're consuming . . . I think I've been in an environment where feelings were so measured. . . . It's almost like a family image that comes to me . . . where things aren't stopped, where they're not repressed. Where they're bountiful. I think my natural exuberance as a child was prohibited. But it's just that letting things tumble out of you in an unrestrained way and letting yourself *be* doesn't mean that horrible things are going to tumble out.

T: But it sounds like the fear is that it's all-consuming and that you don't really know where it's going to lead in a way.

R: Yes.

T: And maybe that's what you mean when you say "It's bigger than the both of us."

R: Yes.

T: Because there's a kind of uncharted territory in a way.

R: Yeah.

T: For me as well. I feel a sense of contact with you right now . . . a sense of connection and intimacy, and there's a sense that the feelings are not something I have control of.

R: Yeah. I think that's it. You've got to keep those reins on. But the idea of it is such a wonderful image for me.

T: Well, I was struck by your words before, "A family image . . . bountiful." There's a real sense of richness there.

R: Yeah.

The final two sessions were devoted to summing up and consolidation. Ruth's feeling was that the seed of a new way of being in relationships was beginning to grow in her. She was able to acknowledge her sadness about separating from the therapist and her anxiety about the future, as well as to express a growing optimism and belief that things could be different in her life. Things had not changed dramatically at work, nor had she gotten into a new romantic relationship. But she felt a subtle sense of beginning to feel more empowered in general and more hopeful about the possibility of things being different for her in intimate relationships. Various strands that emerged in the treatment were never completely tied together, and certain issues were touched on, but not explored in depth. For example, Ruth and her therapist never developed a real understanding of the origin and meaning of her feelings of suffocation in moments of intimacy, and some of her feelings toward the therapist (e.g., sexual feelings) were touched on or alluded to, but not explored in depth. This lack of closure is typical in BRT; learning to live with this type of ambiguity is one of the important lessons for both patients and therapists. This is true in any therapy, but working within a short-term time frame heightens this issue and forces therapists to struggle with their grandiose ambitions and come to terms with their own lack of understanding and control.

In summary, it seems that the first stage in the treatment process entailed the therapist becoming embedded in a relational configuration with Ruth in which her particular way of managing vulnerable feelings and maintaining a safe distance in relationships contributed to his feelings of boredom, disengagement, and frustration. His attempts to disembed from this configuration through metacommunication activated a new cycle of interaction in which her compliance became intensified or at least more salient. His attempt to metacommunicate about this compliance resulted in more compliance, although it may have helped to prepare the ground for her to begin to break out of her compliant stance in subsequent sessions. Although this compliance continued at one level, at another level important progress was being made in terms of Ruth coming to feel more trusting of the therapist and more willing and able to bring her deeper needs and wishes into the relationship.

When she finally did begin to assert herself in relation to the therapist, his ability to survive her aggression without retaliating played a critical role in helping her bring her resentment and dissatisfaction more fully into the relationship. It was at this point that Ruth's awareness of the brief therapy time frame played a pivotal role in accelerating her ability to acknowledge and express her feelings of dissatisfaction with the treatment and her anger and hurt about the therapist's failure to care about her in the way that she desired. This failure of his was expressed in his feelings of irritation, frustration, and boredom with her and in his unwillingness to extend the length of the treatment.

Would it have been more therapeutic for the therapist to silently contain, rather than metacommunicate, his negative feelings toward her? This question seems particularly relevant given the fact that she did find his countertransference disclosure quite hurtful. One cannot rule out the possibility that if he had been able to manage his feelings internally and provided more of a holding en-

vironment, she would have found it helpful. On the other hand, Ruth was particularly sensitive to subtle signs of rejection, and it may have been difficult for the therapist to provide her with the type of authentic caring she needed without first acknowledging what she no doubt perceived implicitly about his attitude (see Bass, 1996). In doing so, he gave her an opportunity to respond with her legitimate feelings of anger and hurt, and this in turn helped the therapist to appreciate her dilemma and to move through his own countertransference feelings and out of his egocentric stance.

A second question that arises is whether it would have been more beneficial for the therapist to extend the time limit once he began to understand how meaningful and important that would have been for her as a tangible act of caring on his part. It seems reasonable to assume that extending the treatment could have been helpful to her and that she could potentially have learned a lesson she was not able to learn from short-term therapy: that it is possible to depend on another person over an extended period of time who is able and willing to be there to the best of his or her ability through both bad and good times. In other words, long-term treatment could have brought about the type of change in her relational schema that would be impossible to effect in short-term treatment. On the other hand, the time-limited nature of the treatment helped Ruth to experience the legitimacy of her needs, in the face of an imperfect world and in a relationship with a therapist who she experienced as "good enough," despite his unwillingness to be there for the long term.

A related question is whether the therapist's unwillingness to extend the time limit constituted a type of retraumatization for Ruth? Is it possible that his terminating at a point when she was beginning to open up and trust was experienced as yet another abandonment in her life? While this possibility cannot be ruled out, Ruth did report finding the treatment helpful, despite the intensity of the conflicting emotions she experienced. We believe that in the final analysis, a critical factor determining whether termination in short-term therapy is experienced as a catalyst for change or a traumatic event is the therapist's ability to process a full range of emotions (both the patient's and his or her own) in a nondefensive fashion. He needs to be able to listen to and accept the patient's anger, disappointment, hurt, and resentment, as well as the gratitude and positive feelings. And he needs to allow himself to experience his own feelings of sadness, disappointment, loss, regret, and guilt, as well as his feelings of warmth, caring, gratification, and pride. In other words, it is critical for therapists not to hide behind theoretical justifications for the time frame, but rather to struggle to meet their patients in an authentic fashion up until the last moment. This involves struggling to understand the unique meaning for them of terminating with each patient, in the same way that they help their patients explore the meaning of termination. It involves struggling with the very questions that we are addressing here. In this way, the time limit can become a catalyst for a true meeting, rather than a barrier.

A Relational Approach
to Training and Supervision

Supervision is central to the training of psychotherapists. And yet, as Martin Rock (1997) puts it, "In spite of its importance, remarkably little attention has been devoted to discussions of the nature of the process and the factors which contribute to its effectiveness or ineffectiveness" (p. 3). This neglect of the topic of training is paralleled in most of the major treatment manuals (e.g., Strupp & Binder, 1984; Luborsky, 1984; Beck, Rush, Shaw, & Emery, 1979; Klerman, Weisman, Rounsaville, & Chevron, 1984). This omission may not be a critical problem when the focus is the acquisition of narrowly defined, concrete technical skills for the treatment of circumscribed problems. If there is one thing that experience has taught us, however, it is that the training of therapists to work skillfully with therapeutic impasses is a formidable task.

The findings of the previously described Vanderbilt II study, conducted by Hans Strupp and his colleagues (see Strupp, 1993), highlight the ambitiousness of this challenge. One of their central objectives was to evaluate the effectiveness of a program for training therapists to work with difficult and potentially pernicious transference–countertransference issues. Recall that in this study experienced psychologists and psychiatrists treated a cohort of patients and then completed a 1-year manualized training program that placed particular emphasis on dealing with maladaptive interpersonal patterns enacted in the therapeutic relationship. They then treated another cohort of patients. Contrary to expectations, the therapists failed to improve in their ability to deal with negative process as a result of the training program; indeed, in some respects they actually deteriorated. There was a tendency for the therapists, following training, to intervene in a forced and mechanical fashion and to act in a more hostile fashion toward their patients (Henry, Strupp, et al., 1993).

How then are we to go about training therapists to deal with the challenge of handling therapeutic impasses and negative therapeutic process? The answer lies in the nature of the skills that we are trying to teach. First, as we have emphasized throughout this book, the relevant skills are not just narrowly defined technical skills: they are also complex, multifaceted inner and interpersonal skills. In order to disembed from enactments, therapists require a basic capacity for self-acceptance (or at least an ability to work toward it), as well as the willingness and courage to face their own demons and to engage in an ongoing process of self-exploration and personal growth. They also require certain basic skills, including interpersonal sensitivity, perceptiveness, and tact, as well as the capacity for intersubjectivity (in the sense of being able to apprehend the patient's perspective and of being able to experience the patient as a subject rather than as an object). Related to this is the capacity to engage in genuine dialogue with the patient, through which therapists are willing to challenge their own preconceptions.

A second important aspect of therapeutic skill is that, like expertise in any field, it has an important intuitive or tacit quality to it. As Dreyfus and Dreyfus's (1986) research on expertise in a variety of different fields shows, unlike beginners, experts do not follow rules or pursue goals in a detached, explicit fashion. Instead, they appraise the situation in a rapid, holistic, and partially automatic fashion. Important aspects of this skill are embodied and tacit. In fact, the explicit, detached following of rules or clear-cut goals can actually interfere with skillful performance.

The cognitive sciences make a distinction between declarative and procedural knowledge that can also help to shed light on the difficulty here (see Binder, 1999). Declarative knowledge is explicit in nature and can be taught in a didactic fashion. In contrast, procedural knowledge is tacit in nature and can only be acquired gradually through real-life experience.

This experience gives individuals an opportunity to apply declarative knowledge in a practical context and to reflect on the consequences. This allows them to modify their declarative knowledge in response to environmental feedback and to develop complex and implicit working models that can guide their actions in ambiguous situations. This type of real-life experience permits skilled therapists to develop complex pattern recognition abilities and the ability to integrate information from multiple sources (e.g., theory, personal affective reactions, patient responses at both verbal and nonverbal levels) in an unconscious fashion.

In addition, skilled psychotherapists, like experts across a range of different domains (e.g., musicians, architects, engineers, managers) develop the ability to *reflect-in-action* (Schon, 1983). This reflection does not necessarily involve conscious mental processing. It is often experienced at a feeling or intuitive level. Nevertheless, it involves a reflective conversation with the relevant situation that allows them to modify their understanding and actions in response to ongoing feedback. It is this type of procedural knowledge in combination with the ability to reflect in action that allows experts to improvise in a fashion that is responsive to the particularities of the moment. This is true whether the case involves a jazz musician creating an innovative riff when jamming with fellow musicians or a therapist responding in a unique way to the relational configuration emerging in the moment with the patient (see Binder, 1999; Safran & Segal, 1990).

What implications do these factors have for the training of therapists? As Hans Strupp and Timothy Anderson (1997) conclude in the wake of the Vanderbilt II Study, while manuals may be of some use in this process, they can never be more than a "useful beginning or a reference" (p. 80). Learning to do therapy is similar to learning any complex skill (and for that matter, similar to personal growth in psychotherapy): it is a complex multidimensional process that includes components such as mentoring, internalization, identification, role modeling, guidance, and socialization.

Training needs to go beyond the didactic presentation of declarative knowledge if therapists are going to develop the combination of procedural knowledge, self-awareness, and reflection-in-action skills necessary to respond to patients in a flexible and creative way. It is important for therapist training to include a substantial experiential component and to emphasize the process of personal growth. As Edgar Levenson (1998) says,

> How do instruction and rules "sink in"? Catching on, "getting it" is an extremely obscure process. It requires translating from a formal set of rules into an experiential grasp. All of us have had the experience, the "ah-hah" phenomenon. "So that's what it feels like" has a very indirect relationship to "this is how to do it." But once one has the feeling, the instructions seem suddenly to have acquired a new clarity. . . . I have the very distinct impression that what trainees need is not a catechism that teaches the relationship of the institute's beloved canons to treat-

ment, but a way of experiencing the analytic process as not so different from the learning of any other skill. There is some common denominator of learning that is prelanguage, almost proprioceptive; perhaps rather than teaching we should be establishing the preconditions for learning. (pp. 247–248)

Below, we discuss a number of ways of establishing these preconditions. They consist of (1) explicitly establishing a focus that privileges the experiential and nonconceptual, (2) using structured mindfulness exercises to help therapists develop the capacity to become observers of their own experience, (3) emphasizing self-exploration and personal growth in the training process, (4) collaboratively exploring the trainee–supervisor relationship for the purposes of working through impasses in the learning process, (5) using audio or video recordings of the treatment, (6) using awareness-oriented role plays for the purposes of heightening therapists' awareness, and (7) modeling therapeutic skills for trainees by giving them an opportunity to observe the supervisor doing therapy (e.g., through observing videotapes of the supervisor doing therapy or observing him or her helping other trainees to explore their own experience in a training group).

EXPLICITLY ESTABLISHING AN EXPERIENTIAL FOCUS

For many trainees, the process of establishing an experiential focus involves a partial unlearning of things that they have already learned about doing therapy. Often the training of therapists emphasizes the conceptual at the expense of the experiential. Trainees study the approaches of different psychotherapy theorists and learn to apply the ideas that they are learning to their clinical experience. They learn how to develop case formulations from different theoretical perspectives and to make interpretations that are guided by their theoretical understanding of what is going on. Although this type of knowledge is essential, it can also serve a defensive function. It can help them to manage the anxiety that inevitably arises as a result of confronting the inherent ambiguity and chaos of lived experience and lead to premature formulations that foreclose experience. It can also help then to avoid dealing with the painful, frightening, conflicting feelings that inevitably emerge for both patients and therapists. On the one hand, this conceptual knowledge can be useful in managing one's anxieties and navigating therapeutic impasses. On the other hand, it can blind therapists to the immediate experience of the moment.

It is useful to begin supervision by explicitly presenting a rationale for emphasizing the experiential in training. We typically begin training by discussing the dangers of reification and emphasizing the value of striving to develop a beginner's mind. We encourage trainees to attempt to relate to videotapes of other trainees' therapy sessions at an experiential level (rather than at a conceptual level) and to give feedback of a more experiential nature. For example, instead of asking our trainees to speculate about the patient's motivation, we encourage them to talk about how they might have felt if they were the therapist or the patient, or to focus on what they are feeling while they are viewing the videotape, or to comment on what is observable (e.g., "You look angry there" or "The patient looks sad to me").

At first, this approach can be difficult for trainees. It is not uncommon for them to respond to questions such as "What are you feeling?" with responses such as "The patient was trying to get a response from me" or "The patient is trying to communicate her own disowned feelings to me." Members of the group can feel strained by focusing on the experiential level, and may complain that the process is artificial and limiting. In response, supervisors can agree that it *is* artificial and limiting to focus on the experiential level at the expense of the conceptual level, but that this is only a stage, until group members find it more natural to focus on the experiential level. Over time, a group culture develops that is more experiential in nature. Then a more natural flow back and forth between experiential and conceptual levels emerges. At first, however, the disciplined and intensive focus on the experiential may feel constraining in the same way that attempting to correct one's overlearned stroke in tennis will feel unnatural.

A useful exercise for purposes of helping trainees begin to distinguish between the experiential and the conceptual (one borrowed from gestalt therapy) consists of having them work in pairs in which they take turns relaying whatever emerges in awareness for them. The other partner is instructed to label each awareness as belonging either to the "inner zone," which includes feelings and physical sensations; to the "outer zone," which consists of immediate perceptions of the outside world; or to the "middle zone," which includes thoughts, inferences, fantasies, and the like. For example, a trainee might say: "Now I'm aware of feeling anxious [inner]. Now I'm aware of the look on your face [outer]. Now I'm aware of how pointless this exercise is [middle]." Although the distinction between these three realms is not always clear, the processes of systematically articulating one's own experience in the here-and-now and of attempting to distinguish between these three realms are useful in terms of helping trainees both to learn to attend to their immediate experience and to distinguish between conceptual and experiential levels.

MINDFULNESS TRAINING

In addition, it can be useful to spend some time talking about the concept of mindfulness and the role that it plays in the therapeutic process. At first, trainees typically have difficulty distinguishing between their experience and their ideas about their experience. Thus it can be useful to use structured mindfulness exercises at the beginning of training in order to help them grasp this distinction and to develop an openness to their experience. Such exercises also help trainees sharpen their abilities to become participant-observers.

One simple exercise, borrowed from Jon Kabat-Zinn (1991), involves instructing trainees to eat a first raisin in a normal fashion and then to eat a second raisin slowly and deliberately while paying careful attention to the entire experience: the taste of the raisin, the feeling of the raisin on the tongue, and so on. This helps them to gain a sense of the distinction between approaching an experience the way we usually do (i.e., mindlessly) and approaching it mindfully.

A second exercise consists of instructing trainees to attend to their bodies for a few moments in an attempt to become aware of any physical sensations that emerge (e.g., itches, tension, restlessness, etc.). During this exercise, they can also be instructed to note when they find their mind wandering away from their physical sensations, in the form of thoughts or fantasies, and then to gently return their attention to their bodies. The first part of the exercise helps them learn to direct their attention and to investigate a specific aspect of their experience (i.e., physical sensations) mindfully. The second part helps them learn to note when their attention is wandering.

A third exercise consists of a more standard mindfulness training. Trainees are instructed to attend to their breaths and to focus on their inhalations and exhalations. When they notice that they are no longer attending to their breaths (as they inevitably will), they are instructed to note what they are attending to instead of their breaths and then to gently return their attention to their breaths. The realization that one is no longer focusing on one's breath thus serves as a cue to note the current focus of one's attention, thereby bringing into awareness that which has been out of awareness, either partially or fully.

For example, I suddenly realize that I am no longer attending to my breath and note that I have been thinking about an appointment I have 2 hours from now. I then gently return my attention to my breath. A few moments later I realize that my attention has wandered from my breath again and note that I have been absorbed in a memory of an argument I had with my wife this morning and that my body is tensing up in anger. I gently return my attention to my breath, where it stays for another few moments. Then I notice that I have forgotten my breath once again and criticize myself for being so easily distracted. If I become absorbed in this self-criticism in a nonmindful fashion, a few moments may pass before I become fully aware of what I am doing to myself. When, however, I do observe this self-criticism directly, it begins to shift my experience of it. It may lighten its intensity. Or I may find myself struggling to push it away. If this is the case, this struggle becomes the focus of observation and investigation. And, as always, I continue to return my attention to my breath as an anchor point.

Trainees are instructed to observe the contents of their awareness without judgment and without letting themselves get caught up in or identified with any particular content of awareness. This involves a conscious effort to "let go" of whatever one's attention has become momentarily absorbed by. This letting go is not the same as suppressing or ignoring; rather, it is a spontaneous dissolving of the momentary focus of attention as a by-product of awareness. Trainees are instructed that the goal is not to eliminate thoughts or feelings, but rather to become more fully aware of them as they emerge on a moment-by-moment basis, without judging them or pushing them away. Gradually, over time, this type of mindfulness work helps trainees to become more aware of subtle feelings, thoughts, and fantasies emerging on the edge of awareness when working with their patients, which can subsequently provide an important source of information about what is occurring in the relationship. One of the most valuable by-products of this kind of mindfulness work is a gradual development of a more tolerant and accepting stance toward a full range of internal experiences.

SELF-EXPLORATION

There are times when specific suggestions about ways of conceptualizing a case or intervening are useful to trainees. Nonetheless, in our approach we emphasize helping trainee therapists to find their own unique solutions to their problems. The particular therapeutic interaction that is the focus of supervision is unique to a particular therapist–patient dyad. Each therapist will thus have her unique feelings in response to a particular patient, and the particular solution she formulates to her therapeutic dilemma must emerge in the context of her own unique reactions. One therapist may respond to a particular patient with a desire to nurture, and another may respond to the same patient with feelings of resentment. The therapist who feels resentment will inevitably have to find some way of working with these feelings, just as the therapist who feels nurturant must begin with these feelings.

Ultimately, both therapists will have to harness whatever feelings they have to be used as part of the therapeutic process.

Therefore, an important focus of training is helping therapists to develop some means of dialoguing with their patients about what is going on in the moment in a way that is unique to the moment and their experience of it. Suggestions about what to say that are provided by supervisors or fellow trainees may look appropriate in the context of a videotape that is being viewed, but may not be appropriate to the context of the next session. The supervisor's task is to help trainees develop the ability to attend to their own experience of the moment and then use it as a basis for intervening. Self-exploration thus plays a central role in supervision.

There has always been a tension between the emphasis on the didactic elements of training, on the one hand, and the self-exploratory and personal growth aspects, on the other. Rock (1997) refers to this as the "teach or treat dilemma." One of the problems with emphasizing the therapeutic aspects of training is that it places the supervisor in a dual relationship with the trainee. On the one hand, the supervisor needs to provide the trainee with the conditions of safety necessary to facilitate his or her self-exploration. On the other hand, he or she is in a position of authority and has an evaluative role. Nevertheless, given the central role that therapists' ability to work with their own inner experience plays in the therapeutic process, it is difficult not to accord a central role to self-exploration in training.

Given the potentially threatening nature of self-exploration for therapists and the complexity of the dual relationship between trainees and supervisors, it is important to pay proper attention to establishing an adequate *supervisory alliance*. The first step in this process consists of explicitly discussing the role that self-exploration plays in training at the outset. In the same way that the establishment of the therapeutic alliance involves both implicit and explicit negotiation of the tasks and goals of treatment, the development of a supervisory alliance involves the negotiation of relevant tasks and goals. It is important for the supervisor to be as clear as possible at the outset of training about the rationale for having an experiential focus to supervision and for emphasizing the central role that self-exploration will play.

When we train therapists in a group context, we typically begin by speaking about the fact that self-exploration will play a central role in supervision and make it clear that we anticipate that some therapists may find that they feel less comfortable with this emphasis than others. We also establish a trial period to give therapists an opportunity to determine whether they feel comfortable with the training approach. We encourage those who find that they do not feel comfortable to leave after this trial period. When we outline the details of this trial period at the beginning, we emphasize that it is not unusual for individuals to find that even though he or she may agree in theory with the importance of self-exploration and working at an experiential level in training, he or she find that the reality of training in this fashion is different from his or her expectations. Thus, it is important to actually have some experience of the training process before committing oneself to it.

We also acknowledge the dual nature of the supervisory relationship at the outset and spend time exploring trainees' concerns about the way in which this dual relationship can make it difficult to feel safe enough to explore feelings, vulnerabilities, and conflicts when they emerge during the training process. We work to establish an agreement in advance that both trainees and supervisors will explicitly discuss any concerns that emerge about the dual nature of their relationship as training proceeds. It is critical for supervisors to understand and acknowledge the realistic dimension of such concerns and to respect trainees' needs to limit self-disclosure to a level that feels comfortable to them at any point in time.

At the outset, we make it clear that while self-exploration plays a central role in the training process, it is also critical for therapists to respect their own needs for privacy and their own fluctuating assessments of what feels safe to explore in front of both supervisors and fellow trainees at any point in time. We thus emphasize that it is important for trainees to monitor their own degree of comfort with self-exploration on an ongoing basis and to take responsibility for halting the exploratory process when they feel uncomfortable with going further. We try to convey to therapists that in supervision, just as in therapy, developing a sense of confidence in one's right to say "No" and one's ability to set personal boundaries (thereby individuating from the other) is a crucial learning experience that overrides the importance of exploring a specific theme at any point in time. We also assure them that as supervisors we will attempt to be respectful of these needs and will try not to push beyond a point that feels right for them in any given context. As training proceeds, we strive to act in a manner that is consistent with this respectful attitude and to be responsive to trainees' feedback that we are pushing too hard. Over time, as therapists come to experience us as trustworthy and respectful of their appropriate needs for privacy, and also come to recognize our earnestness with respect to this, they find it easier to take risks and to explore vulnerable areas. They also find it easier to say "No" and protect their privacy needs.

THE RELATIONAL CONTEXT OF SUPERVISION

In training, as in therapy, the relational context is of utmost importance: it is impossible for the supervisor to convey information to the trainee that has meaning independent of the relational context in which it is conveyed. A series of survey studies (Rock, 1997) have found that good supervisors are experienced by trainees as attuned to their emotional and learning needs. They invite their trainees to identify with them, to take them as mentors, and yet at the same time they encourage autonomy. When things go well, the supervisory relationship is experienced by supervisees as reciprocal, mutual, and trusting. When there is no trust in the supervisory relationship, trainees attempt to conceal their difficulties and countertransferential issues and to present a competent face to supervisors. Supervision can become a process of going through the motions, with trainees striving to deal with what they experience as an assault on their self-esteem and to appear nondefensive, rather than truly learning.

It is important for supervisors to recognize and support trainees' needs to maintain their self-esteem, and to calibrate the extent to which trainees have more of a need for support versus exploration, for new information, or for confrontation in a given moment. It is also important for supervisors to tailor feedback to each trainee's unique needs. Depending where in his or her unique developmental trajectory a particular trainee is, different lessons may be appropriate. For example, for a therapist who feels uncomfortable using countertransference disclosure, experimenting with it can be a worthwhile experience, regardless of the finesse with which it is done. For a therapist who is overly intrusive, the process of sitting back quietly, listening to the patient, and monitoring his own internal processes may be a worthwhile experience.

It is often useful for trainees to begin by articulating the particular issue or theme on which they want to concentrate. In any given session, there are an infinite number of themes on which one can focus. Encouraging trainees to begin by identifying a theme for supervision facilitates the development of the supervisory alliance by increasing the possibility for agreement about supervisory goals. Although the theme may shift over the course of a supervision session, starting with the problem identified by the trainee always provides a useful point of reference. For example, a trainee who begins a supervision session by saying she feels hopeless about working with her patient may need help exploring, accepting, and understanding her feelings of hopelessness more than she needs suggestions about a particular intervention. Similarly, a trainee who comes to supervision looking for confirmation that he is doing a good job, may find suggestions about particular interventions undermining.

When a therapist is troubled by a particular issue and the supervisor or other trainees provide feedback that is irrelevant to this issue, it can be experienced as overwhelming and confusing, rather than as constructive. Assigning trainees the task of articulating a particular theme to work on can be helpful to them in terms of disciplining their sense of focus and establishing a readiness to work. Unless one has defined a problem for oneself, one may have difficulty being open to a solution. Unless one has a question, any answer is meaningless.

It is critical for supervisors to monitor the quality of the supervisory relationship in an ongoing fashion that parallels the ongoing monitoring of the quality of the alliance in therapy. When the alliance is adequate, the supervisory relationship becomes background and does not need to be explicitly addressed. When, however, strains or tensions emerge in the relationship, the exploration of the supervisory relationship should assume priority over all other forms of supervision.

One of the more common frameworks used for thinking about the supervisory relationship is the parallel process model, originally introduced by Harold Searles (1955) and Ekstein and Wallerstein (1958). In this model, the patient's conflicts and defenses are unwittingly enacted by the therapist in supervision, thereby making them available for exploration in an experientially alive fashion. The value of this framework is that it sensitizes supervisors and therapists to potential parallels between scenarios being enacted in both supervisory and therapeutic relationships, and provides a way of harnessing difficulties emerging in the supervisory relationship for purposes of understanding the therapeutic relationship.

The disadvantage of the parallel process framework is that it can function as a reification that provides both supervisor and therapist with a way of distancing themselves from the immediate experience of the difficulty of their own relationship. By conceptualizing a supervisory impasse as a transformation of an impasse in the therapeutic relationship, it decreases the possibility of exploring both therapist and supervisor contributions to the impasse in their own terms in a nuanced fashion. It can thus increase the possibility of therapists and supervisors disowning responsibility for their contributions to the interaction. Since in supervision it is usually the supervisor who identifies the presence of a parallel process, the use of this framework is particularly at risk for providing supervisors with a way of defensively removing themselves from the relational equation.

For these reasons, we tend to apply the parallel process framework to supervision sparingly. Instead, we prefer to explore supervisory impasses in their own terms. As in therapy, this involves a collaborative exploration of both partners' contributions to the impasse. Sometimes there are parallels between impasses emerging both in supervisory and in therapeutic relationships, but sometimes there are not. Regardless of whether the process of unraveling the intricacies of a supervisory impasse sheds immediate light on the case being supervised, the process of working through supervisory impasses provides therapists with valuable experiential learning about the process of working through relational impasses.

Another important point to bear in mind is that when a relationship between impasses in both supervisory and therapeutic relationships emerges, the direction of influence is just as likely to be top down as it is to be bottom up (see Rock, 1997). In the conventional parallel process framework, the assumption is that the therapist triggers an enactment in the supervisory relationship through identification with the patient's conflicts; in other words, the direction of influence is assumed to be bottom up. It is just as common, however, for impasses in the supervisory relationship to translate into impasses in the therapeutic relationship. A therapist who is feeling judged by his supervisor is more likely to feel self-critical with his patients; as the Vanderbilt II study (Henry et al., 1990) has shown, this type of self-criticism is likely to translate into negative therapeutic process. Sometimes the direction of influence is bidirectional. A therapist who is feeling stuck with the patient can become particularly self-critical and defensive in supervision, and this can elicit an unwittingly critical or accusatory response from the supervisor. This, in turn, influences the therapeutic relationship in a negative fashion, which intensifies the therapist's self-criticism and defensiveness in supervision. Some of the most important supervision sessions for therapists are those in which the supervisor is able to help them to become more self-accepting at a time when they are feeling particularly stuck and self-critical.

AUDIO- AND VIDEOTAPING

When supervision is based exclusively on therapists' descriptions of a case, it inevitably misses many of the subtle nuances of what goes on between patients and therapists on a moment-by-moment basis. This problem can be reduced to some extent when therapists take detailed process notes, but even the most detailed process notes are inevitably constructions, and partial representations, based on selective attention.

The use of audio or video recordings of sessions in supervision is a simple and powerful way to provide supervisors with a view of the treatment, which is not filtered through therapists' reconstructions. It also provides therapists with an opportunity to step outside of their immediate participation and to view their own sessions as if they were third-party observers. This process in and of itself can help them to disembed from whatever enactments are being played out.

One useful way of using recordings of therapy sessions in supervision involves stopping the tape at moments when therapists appear to be unwittingly participating in an enactment and then asking them to reconstruct their feelings at the time. This device can help them to become aware of feelings that were dissociated at the time, thereby helping them to disembed. For example, the supervisor may hear irritation or frustration in the therapist's voice in the recorded material despite the fact that the therapist's general description of the session indicates no awareness of such negative feelings. The supervisor stops the tape at a juncture where the irritation is particularly evident and says to the therapist, "Any sense of what you were feeling in that moment?"

During this type of exploration, it is particularly important for the supervisor to assume an empathic, exploratory stance that facilitates the articulation of semi-inchoate experience. Therapists should be encouraged to go beyond simple, one-word responses and to explore the subtle edges of their experience. The task for supervisors is to help trainees get at their unformulated experience (Stern, 1997), unthought known (Bollas, 1987), or felt sense (Gendlin, 1981). It is thus particularly critical for supervisors to create a safe environment or a type of transitional space that encourages therapists to play with the subtle edges of their experience.

When supervision is conducted in a group, it is critical for supervisors to create an atmosphere of trust where self-exploration is valued. Group supervision and case conference formats are particularly conducive to competitive attempts to come up with clever or insightful case formulations. When the objective is to facilitate the type of delicate exploration necessary to get at subtle and often threatening experiences, it is important for supervisors to create an environment in which "not knowing" is valued as much as knowing. One of the most important ways of doing this is through modeling. It is important for supervisors to strive to let go of their own needs to be clever and to have all the answers, and instead to value the process of helping trainees explore their own experience and come up with their own answers.

A second way of using recorded material is for supervisors or group members to provide therapists with subjective feedback about the impact that the patient has upon them. This can help therapists to become aware of dissociated feelings that are being played out in the relationship with the patient. For example, members of a training group may give a therapist feedback that if they were treating her patient they would feel subtly devalued. This feedback may help the therapist to become aware of similar feelings of her own, and this in turn may help her to become aware of the way that she has been acting in a pedantic fashion with the patient in an attempt to convince herself of her own worth and competence as a therapist.

A third approach consists of providing therapists with feedback about what others (the supervisor or group members) observe taking place in the interaction between therapist and supervisor. For example, the supervisor may observe that the patient is acting in a hostile fashion and that the therapist is responding in an overly sweet, saccharine way. Bear in mind that while this type of feedback can be useful, it can be particularly threatening to therapists and should be used judiciously or when there is a particularly solid supervisory alliance and group cohesion.

A fourth approach involves having supervisors imagine that they are in the therapeutic situation and then "think aloud" in an attempt to model the type of internal processes that they might have in a comparable situation. In this approach, the supervisor is not modeling what they might say to the patient, but rather describing his or her own internal processes that are not observable. These include feelings, thoughts, intuitions, internal struggles, and observations about what stands out as figural for them (e.g., the look on the patient's face or a change in her voice tone). This approach gives less experienced therapists a glimpse of the covert processes (or at least the supervisor's construction of them) of a more experienced therapist.

A fifth approach involves identifying interventions that do not appear to have been facilitative and providing the therapist with suggestions for alternative ways of intervening. Although this approach has a place in supervision, we find that it is best to use it sparingly. It can undermine therapists' sense of competence and obstruct their attempts to find their own unique creative ways of responding. Nevertheless, it can play a useful role in certain contexts. A related approach involves encouraging therapists to identify interventions that have been nonfacilitative and then to generate alternative interventions.

AWARENESS-ORIENTED ROLE PLAYS

The use of awareness-oriented role plays can be a particularly valuable tool for grounding the training process at an experiential level and promoting self-awareness in trainees. These consist of having therapists role play a segment of a session that has been problematic, either with the assistance of a training group member who plays the role of patient or therapist, or by playing both roles (alternating back and forth between the role of therapist and patient) themselves. Role plays of this type are particularly useful when there is no recorded material available, but they can also be a useful supplement to supervision making use of recorded material. The goal of this type of exercise or experiment is not so much to practice different ways of intervening as it is to facilitate the exploration of feelings, thoughts, and fantasies relevant to the case that is being focused on. Nevertheless, it can also be an opportunity to experiment with different ways of intervening and exploring feelings that block the ability to intervene in certain ways.

When trainees are playing the roles of both the therapist and the patient, it can be useful to have them switch back and forth between two chairs (using the type of two-chair exercise that is common in gestalt therapy) in order to keep the roles distinct and to heighten their own sense of immersion in whatever role they are playing in the moment. Therapists are encouraged to use whatever they remember from the session as a point of departure, but not to worry about recapturing whatever transpired in a faithful fashion. The goal is to facilitate awareness, rather than to reconstruct a scenario in a precise fashion. At different points during the experiment, the supervisor may encourage the therapist to respond "in role" (either as the therapist or as the patient) in a fashion that feels emotionally plausible in the moment, or to attempt to articulate what he or she feels in a given moment. By directing the therapist's attention inward at opportune moments during the awareness experiment, the supervisor can help her to become aware of feelings that are unconsciously influencing the way she interacts with the patient. Sometimes this awareness in itself can help the therapist and patient to begin to shift out of an impasse.

In other situations, this awareness can provide the therapist with information that he can use for purposes of metacommunication. For example, a female therapist who was working with a successful and wealthy woman from an aristocratic family background was feeling stuck in the treatment and confused about what was going on. While viewing a videotape of a session, the supervisor observed a tendency on the therapist's part to make more interpretations than she usually did and a tendency on the patient's part to respond in a somewhat compliant fashion. He encouraged the therapist to play out a segment of the interaction between her and the patient in supervision, by alternating back and forth between playing herself and the patient. At different points in the exercise, the therapist, while playing the patient's role, acted in subtly competitive and devaluing ways. She repeatedly referred to the therapist by her first name in an overly familiar tone and spoke about ways in which her previous therapist (who had charged a considerably higher fee) had been tremendously helpful to her.

Following such moments, the supervisor would ask the therapist to switch back into the therapist's chair and to either respond to the patient in a fashion that seemed plausible to her or to attempt to put into words what she was feeling. The therapist gradually began to get in touch with an experience of being devalued and of feeling competitive with her patient. The supervisor then encouraged her to enact the process of disclosing these feelings to her patient (whom the therapist imagined to be sitting opposite her in the empty chair) during the awareness experiment. When the therapist tried to do this, she looked tense and uncomfortable to the supervisor. The supervisor then asked her what the experience was like for her. This led to an exploration of her discomfort with acknowledging feelings of competitiveness to herself and others. Further exploration led to a deeper, experientially grounded understanding of the way in which this discomfort had played a role in perpetuating the impasse by making it difficult for the therapist to see her own contribution to it.

A useful variation on this type of awareness experiment involves focusing on a particular therapeutic impasse that a therapist has presented by having different supervision group members take turns playing the role of therapist and patient. This format has a number of advantages. First, it gets all of the supervision group members (not just the therapist who is presenting) actively involved in an experiential mode of learning. Second, it reduces the type of one-upmanship that often takes place when other group members provide the therapist who is presenting with feedback or suggestions about the case. By encouraging other group members to struggle experientially with the presenting therapist's dilemma through creative role plays and awareness experiments, the supervisor increases their empathy for the therapist's dilemma and reduces the type of conceptually driven feedback that is often delivered from a one-up position. This increases the sense of mutuality in the group, as well as the degree of trust, and facilitates the type of genuine self-exploration that is most helpful when therapists are caught in a difficult therapeutic impasse. It also increases the possibility that any feedback that is delivered will be experientially grounded and hence useful to the therapist. In addition, the process of watching colleagues role playing the dilemma that the therapist has brought to the group can sometimes provide the therapist with a new perspective on the impasse.

Finally, by playing the role of their own patients, therapists can sometimes develop an empathic understanding that had previously eluded them of their patients' experience. Alternatively, they may become aware of implicit patient communications that for some reason they had not previously attended to; for example, one therapist might not have been aware of how hostile his patient was acting toward him, or another therapist might not have been aware of her patient's deferential manner.

SUPERVISORS AS MODELS

One of the most valuable learning opportunities for trainees is to see their supervisors in action. In the family therapy tradition, it is common for trainees to have the opportunity of observing their supervisors behind a one-way mirror. But opportunities of this type are more unusual in individual therapy supervision. In the same way that surgeons learn from watching an experienced surgeon operate and dancers are inspired by watching a skilled dancer, therapy trainees can benefit greatly just by observing their supervisors conducting therapy. In typical training programs, most of the opportunities for experiential learning arise from trainees' own experiences as patients. The opportunity to experience what it is like to be in the patient's shoes adds an important experiential dimension to the learning process. Observing one's supervisors in action cannot act as a substitute for this experience. However, observing a skilled therapist in action from the perspective of a third-party observer allows trainees to analyze and make sense of what their supervisor is doing in a way that the embedded perspective of the patient makes more difficult.

In addition, the supervisor who is modeling her therapeutic work has the opportunity to stop at various points along the way and respond to questions regarding her internal processes at critical points. Trainees can ask the supervisor to reconstruct what she was thinking or feeling at relevant points, thereby providing her with an opportunity to articulate tacit processes that might otherwise be difficult to get at. If videotape facilities are available, there is no substitute for observing supervisors in session with their own patients. This, of course, inevitably places supervisors in a somewhat exposed and vulnerable position, but the potential payoffs are well worth the risks.

A further advantage of this format is that it provides trainees with an opportunity to see what a supervisor's work is really like, rather than to imagine some idealized version of it. When trainees have this opportunity to observe their supervisors struggling to help their patients, alternating between moments of skillfulness, clarity, and lucidity, and those of bumbling confusion and bewilderment, it helps them to develop a more self-accepting stance toward themselves in their own struggles as therapists. This helps them to acknowledge the painful and conflicting feelings that inevitably emerge for them while working as therapists, and this in turn helps them to disembed from the enactments that will inevitably be played out with their patients and to work through difficult impasses. This attitude of acceptance also filters down to their feelings toward their patients and helps them to become more tolerant of their limitations and more accepting of the ways in which they are stuck.

A second opportunity for observing their supervisors' clinical work is provided when supervisors help trainees to engage in the process of self-exploration in either individual or group supervision. For example, a trainee feels stuck with a passive–aggressive patient, and a supervisor helps her explore the way in which her own conflicts around aggression make it difficult for her to see the way in which she is contributing to an enactment by unconsciously retaliating through aggressive interpretations. Because of the dual nature of the supervisory relationship, exploratory work of this type is likely to be more limited than it will be in actual therapy. On the other hand, the dual nature of the relationship provides supervisors with the opportunity to stop at various points along the way to make didactic points or to ask trainees if they have any questions or observations. This type of interweaving of exploratory and didactic work can provide a particularly rich learning experience. It can also provide supervisors with a skillful way of titrating the intensity of the exploratory work by introducing a certain degree of intellectual distance when they feel that the exploratory process is moving beyond the boundaries that will feel safe in a training context.

Another important opportunity for observing supervisors working clinically is provided when strains in the supervisory alliance are explored. This exploration can range from simply "checking in" to see how a trainee experiences a supervisor's comment (e.g., when the supervisor has an intuition that the trainee felt criticized) to a more in-depth exploration of full-scale strains or ruptures in the supervisory alliance. For example, the supervisor may experience a trainee as responding in a compliant or deferential fashion to his comments and may decide to initiate an in-depth exploration of what is going on in the relationship. Or he may have the intuition that nothing he says is experienced as helpful by a trainee and decide to explore what is going on in a thorough fashion.

In situations of this type, all the principles that apply to negotiating ruptures of the alliance in therapy also apply, and supervisors must be willing to tolerate whatever negative sentiments are expressed by trainees at such times and to explore their own contributions to the interaction. Once again, given the complexities of the supervisory relationship, supervisors may find it useful at such times to titrate the intensity of the exploration, by stopping the process periodically in order to make a didactic point or to entertain questions by group members. This can introduce a certain degree of intellectual distance when appropriate and help both trainee and supervisor step outside of the interaction.

TRAINING ILLUSTRATION

The following transcript comes from an early group supervision session with a group of therapists who were training to work in the Brief Relational Treatment approach.

> The therapist, Simon, presented a case that made him feel "stuck." He maintained that his patient questioned some of the fundamental premises of the therapy and that he was not sure how to handle it. The patient was a 40-year-old single woman, currently living alone, who was having difficulty establishing and maintaining a romantic relationship. She has a tendency to disown her own needs and feels uncomfortable showing vulnerable feelings. One of her closest friends had recently succumbed to AIDS, and she had been looking after his cat for him. Shortly thereafter, the cat died. As she talked about the cat's death, she began to cry and then began to defend against her sadness.

SIMON (*to supervisor and members of training group*): She began to cry and then tried to get away from the crying very quickly. She moved to a more affectively neutral part of the story and began to talk in a chatty way about friends' explanations for why the cat died and so on. When I tried to explore what leads her to avoid the sad feelings, she started to question the method of what we're doing, and that's really what I'm stuck with. I think she pushed some buttons in me.

SUPERVISOR: Why don't you play a little segment of the session [on the videotape] so the group can get a more nuanced sense of what's going on.

Videotaped Session Segment

SIMON: Let's talk about how come you moved away from the sadness. Is it some sort of numbing? A way to numb yourself and then go on with the story? I don't mean to call it a story. It's something you get comfort from, but I think we're both sitting here and wondering why it happened. What do you think it's about? Why do you choose to tell that part of the story?

PATIENT: I think it's a way of getting away from the pain.

SIMON: It's a way of numbing yourself?

PATIENT: I mean, you know, just about every week I come here, and I cry. I wonder if things will ever get solved.

SIMON: So you're not sure that crying has . . .

PATIENT: I feel I've been depressed for most of my life, and I've cried a lot. I mean, what does that say? What does that solve? What does it do except make you feel a little better because it's a physical release. You know . . . part of my expectation of this therapy . . . I go back to that.

SIMON: What do you mean?

PATIENT: I don't know . . . I need more feedback from you . . . I don't know if we agree about what's important.

SIMON: What's missing for you?

PATIENT: Feedback.

SIMON: About what in particular?

PATIENT: What do you see? What do you think about all this? I don't know. . . . You're the psychologist. [End of Segment]

SUPERVISOR: Okay, Simon, why don't you stop the tape here. (*Pause.*) Any sense of what you're feeling at this moment?

SIMON: I don't know. Confused.

SUSAN: Couldn't it be useful at this point to comment on the way in which she goes on the attack to defend against her vulnerability?

SUPERVISOR: Perhaps. But I think it's important in these situations to remember that with hindsight it can be easy to see how you might have dealt with it. But the issue is that when you're in the situation, you're embedded. You can't see beyond it. I know that when I'm the therapist, when I'm stuck, I'm stuck. And it's often only in retrospect that I can gain some sense of what's going on. What I'm going to suggest is this now. Rather than keeping the focus on Simon, I'd like to give other people the opportunity to start doing some work . . . at least in role-play form. I'm wondering if I can have two volunteers: one to play the patient and one to play Simon.

GEENA: I'll play the patient.

HOWARD: I'll play the therapist.

The supervisor instructs Simon to stop the videotape at a point that he imagines might provide a good point of entry into his experience of having his "buttons pushed" and probes for his experience. Simon, however, is not able to put his feelings into words. At this point, one of the trainees (Susan) attempts to be helpful by suggesting a particular technical strategy (i.e., interpreting the defensive function of the patient's attack). The supervisor, however, is reluctant to go down this path since it shifts the focus away from an experiential level and bypasses the critical step of helping Simon to become more fully aware of the way in which his own feelings may be contributing to the impasse. One possibility might be to continue to help Simon explore his reactions. Sensing that Simon is somewhat stuck, however, and that the group is growing impatient, he encourages more group involvement at an experiential level, by structuring a role-play exercise.

SUPERVISOR: Okay. So here we have an impasse. The patient is pressuring the therapist and saying in a sense, "I'm not getting what I want." And the therapist's task is to try to comment on the interaction in a way that facilitates the therapeutic process. The trick is to try to find some way of talking about what's going on in a way that doesn't mobilize further defensiveness on the patient's part. You're the therapist (*pointing to Howard*), and you're the patient (*pointing to Geena*). So can the two of you reenact a little bit of what we saw in the tape? Howard, I'd like you, as the therapist, with the benefit of hindsight, to try to use your experience to metacommunicate with your patient about what's going on. And Geena, I think it will be important for you in the patient's role to try to get some sense of what it feels like getting this kind of feedback from Howard and to respond in a fashion that is informed by the way you're really feeling in role. So if it feels like a criticism or an insult or whatever, you'll try to respond on that basis.

GEENA: I'm not sure how accurately I can play the patient.

SUPERVISOR: Don't worry about getting it exactly right. Just take a while to get into role. We'll take the episode we watched as a point of departure, but things will take on a life of their own.

GEENA [in role as the patient, to Howard]: Okay. I feel like you ask me a lot of questions, but I don't really get a sense of what the purpose of the questions is. I feel like I want some answers, and it's not clear what this process is all about.

HOWARD [in role as the therapist]: There's something that you're wanting from me that you're not getting?

GEENA [as patient]: Yeah. I mean what's the point? What's the purpose? There are certain things I need to work on, and I feel they're not being addressed here.

HOWARD [as therapist]: I hear that you want some answers . . . and also that you don't see how what we're doing will provide them. I guess my sense is that I'm trying to ultimately give you the answers you want by trying to help you expand your awareness of what you're experiencing right here with me and trying to get a sense of what's happening between us, and we may be sort of disagreeing.

GEENA [as patient]: Well, how will that help me? I don't see how talking about what's happening between us will help me. I mean, it's nice. I like you . . . you're great, you know, but I have other relationships in my life and I don't see the connection.

HOWARD [as therapist]: So you don't see how expanding . . . developing a greater awareness of . . .

GEENA [as patient]: I don't see how my becoming more aware will help. That's for you to tell me. That's why I'm here.

HOWARD (to the group): I don't know what I would do in this situation.

SUPERVISOR: What's happening for you right now?

HOWARD: I'm feeling nailed to the wall, but I'm afraid that if I say that to her, it will just alienate her.

SIMON: Yeah. I know that feeling.

SUPERVISOR: So why don't you try metacommunicating about your dilemma to her?

Through their role play, Geena and Howard are able to reconstruct the situation sufficiently well for Howard to feel stuck. When Howard turns to the group for help, rather than allowing people to respond with suggestions, the supervisor uses Howard's plight as an opportunity to explore the feelings that are emerging. Howard articulates his experience of feeling "nailed to the wall," and this vivid phrase helps Simon to sharpen his own awareness of what his experience of being the therapist is like. The supervisor then encourages Howard to experiment with using this experience as a starting point for metacommunication.

HOWARD [as therapist to Geena as patient]: I feel a little bit like I'm being nailed to the wall. I'm feeling like I don't know how to answer your question. I want to stay with you on this, but I'm not quite sure I know what to say.

GEENA [as patient]: Well, I'd be interested in hearing from your point of view, what you think is important in therapy and what you hope to accomplish (*Long pause . . . Howard looks frustrated.*)

SUPERVISOR (*to Howard*): What's happening for you now?

HOWARD: I'm feeling really stuck. I tried to negotiate a way for myself to sort of be in the room, but it feels like she comes back at me with a rapid-fire question, and I'm stuck again. And I don't want it to be a situation where we keep going back and forth in this way.

SUPERVISOR: It's a real bind. You've tried to talk with her about what's going on, and she's put the pressure back on you again. So where do you go from here? Right?

HOWARD: Right.

SIMON: I didn't metacommunicate as much as Howard did, but my sense is that if I had, the same interaction would have happened, and I would have gotten nailed again.

SUPERVISOR: My suggestion is that in this type of situation, you just continue to comment on the process.

HOWARD: Comment on the process?

SUPERVISOR: For example, let's imagine that it keeps going back and forth for a while. I could imagine myself saying something like "I keep trying to put the ball in your court and you keep trying to put it back into mine."

The supervisor uses this role play as an opportunity to help trainees begin to develop an understanding of the importance of continuing to play the role of the participant-observer by noting and commenting on whatever emerges in the moment, rather than becoming fixated on their initial understanding of the situation.

ANDREW: Also, when you say, "I feel nailed to the wall," maybe there's somewhat of a blaming quality to it, that gets her to react defensively. Sometimes, when you're metacommunicating, you think you've broken out of the cycle, but you're actually still caught in it.

SUPERVISOR: Andrew's point is a good point, but it's also important not to take from that the idea that therefore one shouldn't continue to be stuck. The issue is that you're going to be stuck, and that's just part of the process.

HOWARD: Right.

SUPERVISOR: You with me?

HOWARD: Yeah

SUPERVISOR: Okay. Let's have some other people playing these roles.

NICOLE: I'm willing to play the patient.

SUPERVISOR: Okay. Who's willing to play the therapist's role? (*Extended silence and then laughter among group members.*)

SUPERVISOR: Okay. No takers? How come?

JENNIFER: Too hard.

DAVID: The same thing that happens to me in session. My brain freezes. It just freezes up. I don't have the faintest idea of what I could say to get myself out of this.

SUSAN: Right. Frozen under the spotlight.

SUPERVISOR: Okay. Now in some ways this is perhaps more difficult than an actual session, because there's the additional factor of the stage fright. But there's another way in which the pressure you experience here is a good analogue to the pressure you can experience as therapists in this treatment project. We're working with difficult patients, and there are going to be a lot of difficult impasses, and a certain pressure we'll all feel to perform. So I guess I really want to encourage people to get in here, take risks, and screw up. I think it's really important to have that experience of screwing up here in supervision and when you're doing therapy as well.

HOWARD: I want to say something for following in my footsteps. It felt like a good learning experience for me, but it's also validating to see how people aren't rushing to sit in the therapist's chair. My worst fantasy is that you'll all sit in that chair and know exactly what to say.

SUSAN: No way.

SUPERVISOR: It's always easier for people to be backseat therapists and say, "I would have said this" or "I would have said that."

VOICES FROM THE GROUP: Right. Right.

This is an early session for this particular training group and the establishment of a solid supervisory alliance and sense of group cohesiveness is still very much in process. It is not unusual for trainees at first to shy away from taking the kind of risks that role playing and self-exploration require. The supervisor is trying to lay the groundwork for the development of a group culture that prizes openness and the willingness to experiment and take risks, rather than having the "right answers."

SUPERVISOR: Okay. So let's get into role again. Who's willing to play the therapist?

SIMON: Okay . . . I'd like to try.

SUPERVISOR: Okay. So let's get into role.

SIMON: Should we continue where we left off? I'm not sure I can remember. I feel like I have to start at a new point.

SUPERVISOR: That's fine.

SIMON [as therapist]: So tell me what you were saying before about the questions? I want to get a better understanding of what you're feeling in terms of questioning and wanting answers.

NICOLE [as patient]: I just want answers from you. I want some kind of feedback that's going to change the way I've been screwing up my life.

SIMON [as therapist]: Right. . . . What are you feeling right now?

NICOLE [as patient]: Another feeling question. I'm feeling like this just isn't getting me anywhere.
  (*Simon shrugs and gestures to group as if to say "I'm stuck." There is silence for a moment, and then everyone laughs.*)

JENNIFER: Now you know why we didn't want to play the therapist.

SUPERVISOR (*to Simon*): What are you experiencing?

SIMON: I don't know. I just don't have a comeback.

SUPERVISOR: Okay. So you're at a loss.

SIMON: Yeah.

SUPERVISOR: Okay. So can you work from this point? "I'm at a loss" . . . or whatever . . . in other words . . . try to put into words the feeling of the gesture you made to the group.

SIMON: Okay. I don't want to say "I'm at a loss." But let me see . . .

SUPERVISOR: Why not?

SIMON: Well . . . okay. I'll try it.

SUPERVISOR: You don't have to try it . . . but I'm just curious to find out what your reservations are.

SIMON: Well . . . I think of saying, "I don't know," and my heart starts beating.

SUPERVISOR: Can you say a little more?

SIMON: Well . . . it's like my competency is on the line. I guess it feels like that a lot with her.

SUPERVISOR: So it's not okay with you not to have the answers right now?

SIMON: I guess not.

Through the role play Simon accesses an experience of "being at a loss." When the supervisor encourages him to use this experience as a point of departure for metacommunication, Simon contacts some anxiety. He is about to push through this anxiety in an act of compliance, but the supervisor instead uses the opportunity to begin to explore an internal conflict that may be contributing to the therapeutic impasse.

SUPERVISOR: Okay . . . I'm going to suggest an experiment. It sounds like there's an internal split. It's not just that you feel at a loss, but also that there's a part of you that finds that unacceptable. Does that fit?

SIMON: Yeah.

SUPERVISOR: Okay. So can you sit in this chair (*pulls up an empty chair*), and play the part of yourself that finds it unacceptable? (*Simon moves to empty chair.*) . . . In other words, tell the part of you that feels at a loss (*gestures to empty chair*) that it's not acceptable.

SIMON (*speaking to empty chair*): You should have the answers. What's wrong with you? (*Pause.*)

SUPERVISOR: Can you switch to the other chair and respond?

SIMON (*switching to other chair*): I don't know. I guess I'm feeling stuck.

SUPERVISOR: Can you switch chairs and speak as the other side?

SIMON (*switching chairs*): That's not good enough. You should have the answers.

SUPERVISOR: Switch please.

SIMON (*switching chairs*): Well, I don't, and that's all there is to it (*gesturing with hand*).

SUPERVISOR: What's the feeling that goes with the gesture?

SIMON: It's like "Back off. I can't be where I'm not."

SUPERVISOR: Switch chairs please.

SIMON: (*Switches chairs and looks at empty chair thoughtfully.*)

SUPERVISOR: What's happening for you?

SIMON: Well . . . that makes sense. I feel a sense of letting go.

SUPERVISOR: Okay. So now I'm going to suggest as an experiment that you try talking about your feeling of being stuck to your patient and see how it feels. Imagine that she's sitting in the empty chair (*gesturing to it*), and try talking with her about your experience.

SIMON (*to empty chair*): You know ... I'm feeling kind of stuck right now. I'd like to say something that's helpful to you, but I just can't seem to find the right thing to say (*long pause*).

SUPERVISOR: What does that feel like?

SIMON: It actually feels okay. It feels like a relief.

SUPERVISOR: Okay. Now there's no guarantee as to how your patient would respond if you said that ... but it seems like an important place to come to internally.

SIMON: Yeah. I agree.

The supervisor uses a two-chair exercise to help Simon explore the way in which his intolerance of his own feelings of helplessness contributes to the impasse. Because of this intolerance he is more likely to get into a struggle with the patient in an attempt to manage his own feelings of discomfort. By separating out two different parts of the self (i.e., the part that feels helpless and the part that criticizes this part), he becomes more aware of this internal conflict and develops an experiential awareness of the impact of being the object of his own self-criticism. This initiates a process of self-acceptance. This process begins when the part of the self that has been the object of the self-criticism asserts itself and defends itself against the self-criticism ("Back off. I can't be where I'm not."). It continues with a softening of the part of the self that is being critical ("Well ... that makes sense. I feel a sense of letting go.") (Greenberg et al., 1993; Greenberg & Safran, 1987). Although we have abbreviated the transcript somewhat at this point in order to make it more "user-friendly," it still captures the essence of the process through which the shift takes place. This type of internal shift will not be permanent, but it does provide Simon with a momentary taste of what it is like to be more self-accepting on this issue.

NICOLE: I can imagine that if I were the patient I would feel something shift.

JENNIFER: I would be afraid that if I said something like that to my patient, then she would feel abandoned by me.

SUPERVISOR: Okay ... so it's important for you to be aware of that fear. Just like it's important for Simon to recognize that his sense that he needs to be competent makes it difficult for him to tolerate his feelings of helplessness. Whether you actually say something to your patient about your feelings is another question. But the first step is to be able to accept the fact that at times we all feel helpless and hopeless as therapists. And that's part of the process. And somehow we struggle to maintain some kind of faith that if we stick with it, we'll be able to work things out. And I think that if we can try to hold on to that larger picture, some of that will come across to our patients.

SUSAN: But isn't it ultimately important for her to see how she defends herself against her feelings and closes down?

SUPERVISOR: Maybe . . . but remember that your attempts to help her see that may be, at least in part, another move in a struggle that the two of you are locked into.

SUSAN: But I think that exploring her need to defend herself could also be a way of stepping out of the game.

SUPERVISOR: Maybe. You'd have to try it and see. I think in the final analysis the only way you're going to know is on the basis of what happens. It's gonna come down to the patient's experience. If she experiences whatever you do as another attempt on your part to win the game, then you'll stay stuck. If she experiences it as something different, then things may shift. Ultimately, you just do whatever works. You may make what you think is the most brilliant intervention, and if it doesn't work, then you just sort of stumble along until you find something that does. And bear in mind that there's no one solution. And different things will work for different therapists.

Afterword

Over the years various questions have been raised in response to the approach we have presented in this book. In this afterword, we will consider some of the most common ones. We are often asked whether the approach is useful primarily for purposes of dealing with therapeutic impasses or whether it constitutes a more general approach to psychotherapy. Our impression is that, while the principles that we have spelled out are particularly useful for purposes of dealing with ruptures in the therapeutic alliance, they also constitute a useful orientation toward psychotherapy in general. Some of the basic notions, such as the importance of understanding things from the perspective of a two-person psychology, the recognition of our inevitable embeddedness in the interactive matrix, dialectical constructivism, mindfulness, acceptance, attempting to process one's own feelings nondefensively, and the recognition that all interventions are relational acts, seem to us to be valuable principles to keep in mind whether there is currently a strain in the alliance or not.

The therapist, of course, spends less time explicitly addressing the therapeutic relationship when things are running smoothly. At such times, other therapeutic tasks may become foreground (these tasks will vary depending on the therapist's orientation), but the underlying principle of attempting to understand what is being enacted relationally between therapist and patient on an ongoing basis remains important, even if it is not talked about explicitly and assumes a background position. Moreover, one must keep in mind that ruptures in the therapeutic alliance take place more commonly than many therapists realize. Our research program indicates that it is rare to have more than a session or two without some minor strain in the alliance, and that therapists often fail to see ruptures experienced by patients. While it is not critical for the therapist to address every strain explicitly, his or her attentiveness to ongoing fluctuations in the quality of relatedness can open up valuable opportunities for exploration that might not otherwise emerge.

A related question we are asked is whether the approach is useful for all patients or only for those patients with sufficient resources and ego strength to make use of therapeutic metacommunication. We wish to stress that we do not see metacommunication as the essence of the approach we have described. Metacommunication is one particular way of working that grows naturally out of the more fundamental principles of the approach. Sometimes, with some patients, metacommunication can be particularly useful for purposes of disembedding from a relational configuration that is being unwittingly enacted, but other times the process of explicitly trying to clarify what is transpiring in the therapeutic relationship can be experienced as too threatening or impinging. While metacommunication may not be useful with *all* patients or in *all* contexts with a particular patient, we nonetheless believe that the more basic principles we have outlined are generalizable to a fairly broad range of patients. Having said this, we also want to emphasize that in our experience many therapists have a tendency to underestimate patients' ability to make use of metacommunication in a constructive fashion. It is important to differentiate between when therapists are avoiding exploring what is transpiring in the here-and-now of the therapeutic relationship because of an accurate assessment of their patients' sensitivities and limitations and when they do so because of their own anxieties, conflicts, and discomfort with certain aspects of their experience.

It is also important to recognize that different therapists have different personal sensitivities or styles that predispose them to gravitate toward one type of therapeutic stance and to feel less comfortable with other stances (Aron, 1999; Greenberg, 1995). We all have complex and conflicting feelings concerning issues such as self-disclosure, intimacy, and power, and these feelings will necessarily color our relationship to a therapeutic stance that involves metacommunication, countertransference disclosure, or any type of intensive focus on the here-and-now of the therapeutic relationship. They will also color the way our stance is experienced by our patients. As Aron (1999) points out, the relationship between our personal styles and the therapeutic stances we prefer is not always a simple one. One therapist may feel less comfortable with metacommunication because of a more generalized discomfort with all forms of self-disclosure. Another may gravitate toward a more intensive here-and-now focus on the therapeutic relationship in partial compensation for a more private, distant interpersonal style in daily life. One therapist may feel uncomfortable with an emphasis on the mutuality of the therapeutic relationship because of a more generalized need for control. Another may gravitate toward a more mutual and symmetrical stance because of anxieties about assuming the role of the authority. Some therapists are reluctant to focus on the here-and-now of the therapeutic relationship because of their own concerns about intrusiveness. Others have a compulsive need to metacommunicate because of their own difficulty in tolerating anxiety stemming from any uncertainty about what is transpiring in relationships. Our point is that it is difficult to consider the question of whether therapeutic metacommunication will be helpful for a particular patient without first considering the therapist's relationship to the intervention.

Keeping this qualification in mind, it is still worth considering the question of whether the type of intensive focus on the here-and-now of the therapeutic relationship emphasized in this book has associated risks. *Any* intervention or relational stance has inherent risks. Just as definitively offered interpretations or rational challenges to patients' catastrophic expectations are more likely to be experienced as patronizing than are empathic reflections, therapeutic metacommunication has certain inherent properties that can lead to certain types of problems. These will, of course, be mediated by the personal qualities of the therapist, the way in which the metacommunication is expressed, and the unique sensitivities of the patient. One patient may experience an attempt at metacommunication as a form of persecution. Still another may experience the therapist's self-disclosure as a form of narcissistic self-absorption. Another may experience it as impinging or intrusive. All of these experiences may be understandable reactions to the therapist's contribution. In many cases, however, ongoing collaborative exploration can clarify the meaning of the therapist's intervention to the patient. This can facilitate a disembedding from the relational configuration that is being enacted, a greater awareness of the way the therapist is contributing to it, and a deeper understanding of the patient's idiosyncratic sensitivities.

In some cases, however, this disembedding does not take place, and any attempt to further explore the interaction constitutes an intensification of a toxic cycle that is being enacted. In such situations, the therapist may need to step back and use one of the more indirect approaches to impasse resolution described in the taxonomy outlined in Chapter 1. The therapist may, for example, need to *change the therapeutic task* by focusing on out-of-session events and confining him- or herself to responding in an empathic fashion. Other patients may respond better to a more interpretive approach or may need the therapist to provide direct advice or to assume a more active problem-solving stance. If the therapist is able to demonstrate this type of flexibility, the patient may at some later point in time feel sufficiently trusting to explore what is going on in the therapeutic relationship itself. This type of change in the therapeutic task can help to provide the patient with a *new relational experience*.

When therapeutic metacommunication is not an option, it becomes critical for therapists to struggle with and process their own conflicting feelings in a nondefensive fashion, while refraining from explicitly sharing certain aspects of their subjective experiences with the patient. Although at various points in this book we have touched upon the importance of being able to provide this type of holding or containing environment for patients, we have devoted relatively less attention to the question of how to do it than we have to describing interventions that directly and explicitly explore the therapeutic relationship. Just as one cannot simultaneously see the vase and the profiles in the old gestalt figure–ground illustration, it is inevitable that an emphasis on one aspect of therapeutic process will relegate other equally important aspects to the background.

In a recent paper, Greenberg (1999) criticizes what he considers an excess in contemporary relational thinking in the direction of too much emphasis on intersubjective confrontation, therapist self-disclosure, and spontaneity. He argues that many of the published clinical examples share a narrative style in which the therapist responds to a therapeutic impasse by "throwing away the book" and responding in a spontaneous, self-disclosive or personally expressive fashion. While recognizing the value of this type of emphasis, he points out the dangers of neglecting the importance of a more disciplined, self-restrained stance on the therapist's part that can provide patients with the space necessary to engage in their own self-exploration.

Our response to this critique is mixed. On the one hand, we feel it is important to point out that many of the seminal relational thinkers (e.g., Aron, 1996; Hoffman, 1998; Mitchell, 1988) are struggling with the whole issue of the dialectical relationship between ritual and spontaneity (to use Irwin Hoffman's phrase) in a careful and sophisticated fashion, and that it is unfair to accuse them of emphasizing personal responsiveness and spontaneity at the expense of theoretically guided restraint or of emphasizing interpersonal encounter at the expense of a careful, private reflective process. On the other hand, it is true that relatively little attention is devoted in the literature to explicating and illustrating the processes through which therapists can work with their

unpleasant, painful, or interpersonally disjunctive feelings in a constructive fashion during those periods when explicitly hearing about
them will be experienced as impinging by patients. Slochower (1997)
has made a valuable contribution to the relational discourse by emphasizing the potential importance of holding or containment in this type
of context. It is noteworthy, however, that while she argues for the importance of the therapist struggling to fully experience and contain
such feelings, she does not really elaborate on the nature of the internal processes that can help him or her to do this.

What exactly is the nature of the state of mind that allows one to
relate to a difficult, painful, or potentially disjunctive internal experience, without defining oneself by it and without trying to push it away
through a dissociative process or through modulating it by acting (by
either discharging one's feeling through unwitting action or attempting to metacommunicate about it in a more reflective fashion)? How
can we begin to talk about it and how do we enter into it? Bromberg
(1996, 1998), for example, refers to this experience as one of "standing
in the spaces," by which he means that one is able to "make room at any
given moment for subjective reality that is not readily containable by
the self he experiences as 'me' in the moment" (Bromberg, 1996, p.
516). He invokes the metaphor of "playing" in an attempt to capture an
aspect of this experience. The notion of playing *does* seem to capture
something important about the experience in at least two respects.
First, it has the connotation of a certain lightness about it, as opposed
to the heaviness of feeling completely defined by a particular self-state,
or of struggling not to be so. Second, playing has the quality of being
unbidden or unwilled. This seems critical as well. The state of mind
that we are trying to point at has a quality of surrender to it. We cannot
will ourselves into accepting. We all know what this experience of "letting go" is like. For example, you're walking along the street tied up in
knots both emotionally and physically as you dwell on a painful experience, perhaps a significant loss or a disappointment. Suddenly, you
hear the strains of a familiar tune playing on the radio—a sad song that
resonates with your feelings. You begin to experience the knots unty-
ing, something flows more freely inside you, and your relationship to
your pain begins to shift. You are now both experiencing the pain and
observing yourself in the process of experiencing it. The internal struggle may not disappear completely, but it becomes less intense, or its intensity ebbs and flows, and you are able to observe this ebb and flow as
well. We all know what this experience is like, yet how can it be cultivated if the very act of trying to do so can get in the way?

One of the problems in talking about this type of process is that it
is intrinsically more difficult to write about our own internal processes,

both in terms of the willingness to reveal private material and in terms of the ability to reconstruct subtle and fleeting internal processes. Writers such as Ogden (1994) and Jacobs (1991) provide interesting models of the way in which this type of writing can be done. Each has his own unique characteristic focus of self-exploration and style of writing. Ogden tends to reconstruct his own fleeting moment-by-moment associations to the patient's material. In many cases, these associations initially seem meaningless or irrelevant to the clinical issue at hand, but he subsequently constructs meaning out of them and uses this process to guide his interpretive activity. In contrast, Jacobs tends to focus on personal memories (often from the distant past), emotions, and self-states that in some way resonate with aspects of the patient's dynamics, and uses this type of reflection to deepen his understanding of these dynamics. His style of self-reflection tends to have less of an immediate, moment-by-moment quality to it, but in some respects is more personal or self-revealing. Taken together, their work provides hints of a new, potentially fruitful type of narrative genre that could be further developed.

Another potentially productive direction involves integrating mindfulness practice or some variant of it into the training of psychotherapists in a more systematic and disciplined fashion. In the Zen tradition, there is a saying that "reading about Zen is like counting another man's cows." One can benefit from familiarizing oneself with the philosophy and principles of mindfulness and attempting to integrate them into one's practice as a psychotherapist, but it is not quite the same as setting aside a regular time for sitting and looking at one's own mind in a disciplined fashion.

The psychoanalytic tradition assumes that the development of the capacity for self-observation is critical for the skilled therapist. Aside from the requirement that therapists undergo a personal analysis, however, there is nothing built into the training model to increase the possibility that therapists maintain and refine whatever capacity for self-observation they have developed, on an ongoing basis over time. Of course, one could argue that the ongoing practice of psychotherapy in a self-reflective fashion, combined with peer supervision or discussion with one's colleagues, is a form of mindfulness practice in itself. But is this the same as cultivating a formal mindfulness practice? This is where our book ends, but, we hope, not the conversation.

References

Alexander, F. (1948). *Fundamentals of psychoanalysis*. New York: Norton.

Alexander, F., & French, T. M. (1946). *Psychoanalytic therapy*. New York: Ronald Press.

Alexander, L. B., & Luborsky, L. (1986). The Penn helping alliance scales. In L. S. Greenberg & W. M. Pinsof (eds.), *The psychotherapeutic process: A research handbook* (pp. 325–366). New York: Guilford Press.

Arnkoff, D. (1995). Two examples of strains in the therapeutic alliance in an integrative cognitive therapy. *In Session: Psychotherapy in Practice, 1*, 33–46.

Aron, L. (1996). *A meeting of minds: Mutuality in psychoanalysis*. Hillsdale, NJ: Analytic Press.

Aron, L. (1998). Clinical choices and the theory of psychoanalytic technique: Commentary on Mitchell's and Davies' papers. *Psychoanalytic Dialogues, 8*, 207–216.

Aron, L. (1999). Clinical choices and the relational matrix. *Psychoanalytic Dialogues, 9*, 1–29.

Aron, L., & Harris, A., eds. (1991). *The legacy of Sandor Ferenczi*. Hillsdale, NJ: Analytic Press.

Atwood, G., & Stolorow, R. (1984). *Structures of subjectivity: Explorations in psychoanalytic phenomenology*. Hillsdale, NJ: Analytic Press.

Bacal, H. A., & Newman, K. M., eds. (1990). *Theories of object relations: Bridges to self psychology*. New York: Columbia University Press.

Bach, S. (1985). *Narcissistic states and the therapeutic process*. New York: Aronson.

Bach, S. (1994). *The language of perversion and the language of love*. Northvale, NJ: Aronson.

Bakan, D. (1966). *The duality of human existence*. Boston: Beacon Press.

Baldwin, M. (1992). Relational schemas and the processing of social information. *Psychological Bulletin, 112*, 461–484.

Balint, M. (1968). *The basic fault*. London: Tavistock.

Balint, M., Ornstein, P., & Balint, E. (1972). *Focal psychotherapy*. London: Tavistock.

Barlow, D. (1996). The effectiveness of psychotherapy. *Clinical Psychology: Science and Practice, 3*, 236–240.

Bass, A. (1996). Holding, holding back, and holding on. *Psychoanalytic Dialogues, 6*, 361–378.

Beck, A. T., Rush, J., Shaw, B., & Emery, G. (1979). *Cognitive therapy of depression*. New York: Guilford Press.

Beebe, B., & Lachmann, F. (1992). The contribution of mother–infant mutual influence to the origins of self- and object representations. In N. J. Skolnick & S. C. Warshaw (eds.), *Relational perspectives in psychoanalysis* (pp. 83–118). Hillsdale, NJ: Analytic Press.

Benjamin, J. (1988). *The bonds of love*. New York: Pantheon Books.

Benjamin, J. (1990). An outline of intersubjectivity: The development of recognition. *Psychoanalytic Psychology, 7*, 33–46.

Bernstein, R. (1983). *Beyond objectivism and relativism*. Philadelphia: University of Pennsylvania Press.

Bibring, E. (1937). The results of psychoanalysis. *International Journal of Psycho-Analysis, 18*, 170–189.

Binder, J. L. (1999). Issues in teaching and learning time-limited psychodynamic psychotherapy. *Clinical Psychology Review, 19*, 705–719.

Binder, J. L., & Strupp, H. H. (1997). "Negative process": A recurrently discovered and underestimated facet of therapeutic process and outcome in the individual psychotherapy of adults. *Clinical Psychology: Science and Practice, 4*, 121–139.

Bion, W. R. (1959). Attacks on linking. *International Journal of Psycho-Analysis, 40*, 308–315.

Bion, W. R. (1962). *Learning from experience*. New York: Basic Books.

Bion, W. R. (1967). Notes on memory and desire. In E. B. Spillius (ed.), *Melanie Klein today* (Vol. 2, pp. 17–21). London: Routledge.

Bion, W. R. (1970). *Attention and interpretation*. London: Heinemann.

Blatt, S. J., & Blass, R. B. (1992). Relatedness and self-definition: Two primary dimensions in personality development, psychopathology, and psychotherapy. In J. Barron, M. Eagle, & D. Wolitsky (eds.), *Interface of psychoanalysis and psychology* (pp. 399–428). Washington, DC: American Psychological Association Books.

Bollas, C. (1987). *The shadow of the object: Psychoanalysis of the unthought known*. New York: Columbia University Press.

Bordin, E. (1979). The generalizability of the psychoanalytic concept of the working alliance. *Psychotherapy: Theory, Research, and Practice, 16*, 252–260.

Bordin, E. (1994). Theory and research in the therapeutic working alliance: New directions. In A. O. Horvath & L. S. Greenberg (eds.), *The working alliance: Theory, research, and practice* (pp. 13–37). New York: Wiley.

Bowlby, J. (1969). *Attachment and loss: Vol. 1. Attachment*. New York: Basic Books.

Bowlby, J. (1973). *Attachment and loss: Vol. 2. Separation, anxiety, and anger*. New York: Basic Books.

Bowlby, J. (1980). *Attachment and loss: Vol. 3. Loss: Sadness and depression.* New York: Basic Books.

Bowlby, J. (1988). *A secure base.* New York: Basic Books.

Brenner, C. (1979). Working alliance, therapeutic alliance, and transference. *Journal of the American Psychoanalytic Association, 27,* 137–158.

Breuer, J., & Freud, S. (1893–1895/1955). Studies on hysteria. In J. Strachey (ed. and trans.), *The standard edition of the complete psychological works of Sigmund Freud* (Vol. 2, pp. 1–31). London: Hogarth Press.

Briggs, J. (1988). *Fire in the crucible: The alchemy of creative process.* New York: St. Martin's Press.

Bromberg, P. M. (1993). Shadow and substance: A relational perspective on clinical process. *Psychoanalytic Psychology, 10,* 147–168.

Bromberg, P. M. (1995). Resistance, object-usage, and human relatedness. *Contemporary Psychoanalysis, 31,* 173–191.

Bromberg, P. M. (1996). Standing in the spaces: The multiplicity of self in the psychoanalytic relationship. *Contemporary Psychoanalysis, 32,* 506–535.

Bromberg, P. M. (1998). *Standing in the spaces: Essays on clinical process, trauma, and dissociation.* Hillsdale, NJ: Analytic Press.

Buber, M. (1923/1958). *I and thou* (2d ed., trans. R. G. Smith). New York: Scribner.

Buber, M. (1936/1947). *Between man and man* (trans. R. G. Smith). London: Routledge & Kegan Paul.

Busch, F. (1995). *The ego at the center of clinical technique.* Northvale, NJ: Aronson.

Carpy, D. V. (1989). Tolerating the countertransference: A mutative process. *International Journal of Psycho-Analysis, 70,* 287–294.

Chused, J. (1991). The evocative power of enactments. *Journal of the American Psychoanalytic Association, 39,* 615–640.

Coady, N. (1991). The association between client and therapist interpersonal processes and outcomes in psychodynamic psychotherapy. *Research on Social Work Practice, 1,* 122–138.

Coyne, J., & Pepper, C. (1998). The therapeutic alliance in brief strategic therapy. In J. D. Safran & J. C. Muran (eds.), *The therapeutic alliance in brief psychotherapy* (pp. 147–169). Washington, DC: American Psychological Association Books.

Curtis, H. (1979). The concept of the therapeutic alliance: Implications for the "Widening scope." *Journal of the American Psychoanalytic Association, 27,* 159–192.

Cushman, P. (1995). *Constructing the self, constructing America.* Reading, MA: Addison-Wesley.

Damasio, A. R. (1994). *Descartes's error: Emotion, reason, and the human brain.* New York: Grosset/Putman.

Davanloo, H., ed. (1980). *Short-term dynamic psychotherapy.* New York: Aronson.

Davies, J. M. (1996). Linking the "pre-analytic" with the post-classical: Integration, dissociation, and the multiplicity of unconscious processes. *Contemporary Psychoanalysis, 32,* 553–576.

Dickes, R. (1975). Technical considerations of the therapeutic and working alliances. *International Journal of Psychoanalytic Psychotherapy, 14,* 1–24.

Dinnerstein, D. (1976). *The mermaid and the minotaur.* New York: Harper & Row.

Dreyfus, H. E., & Dreyfus, S. L. (1986). *Mind over machine.* New York: Free Press.

Eagle, M. (1984). *Recent developments in psychoanalysis.* New York: McGraw-Hill.

Ehrenberg, D. (1992). *The intimate edge.* New York: Norton.

Ekman, P. (1993). Facial expression and emotion. *American Psychologist, 48,* 384–392.

Ekman, P., & Davidson, R. J., eds. (1994). *The nature of emotions: Fundamental questions.* New York: Oxford University Press.

Ekstein, R., & Wallerstein, R. (1958). *The teaching and learning of psychotherapy.* New York: International Universities Press.

Eliot, T. S. (1963). *Collected poems, 1909–1962.* New York: Harcourt, Brace & World.

Epstein, L. (1977). The therapeutic function of hate in the countertransference. *Contemporary Psychoanalysis, 13,* 442–468.

Epstein, L. (1979). The therapeutic use of countertransference data with borderline patients. *Contemporary Psychoanalysis, 15,* 248–275.

Epstein, M. (1995). *Thoughts without a thinker.* New York: Basic Books.

Fairbairn, W. R. D. (1952). *Psychoanalytic studies of the personality.* London: Tavistock/Routledge & Kegan Paul.

Farber, L. H. (1966). *The ways of the will: Essays toward a psychology and psychopathology of will.* New York: Basic Books.

Fenichel, O. (1941). *Problems of psychoanalytic technique.* New York: Psychoanalytic Quarterly.

Ferenczi, S. (1915/1980). Psychogenic anomalies of voice production. In J. Richman (ed.), *Further contributions to the problems and methods of psychoanalysis* (pp. 105–109, trans. E. Mosbacher). London: Karnac Books.

Ferenczi, S. (1931/1980). Child analysis in the analysis of adults. In M. Balint (ed.), *Final contributions to the problems and methods of psychoanalysis* (pp. 126–142, trans. E. Mosbacher). London: Karnac Books.

Ferenczi, S. (1932/1988). *The clinical diary of Sandor Ferenczi* (ed. J. Dupont, trans. M. Balint & N. Z. Jackson). Cambridge, MA: Harvard University Press.

Ferenczi, S. (1933/1980). Confusion of tongues between adults and the child. In M. Balint (ed.), *Final contributions to the problems and methods of psycho-analysis* (pp. 156–167, trans. E. Mosbacher). London: Karnac Books.

Ferenczi, S., & Rank, O. (1925/1956). *The development of psychoanalysis.* New York: Dover.

Fiscalini, J. (1988). Curative experience in the analytic experience. *Contemporary Psychoanalysis, 24,* 105–142.

Fonagy, P., & Target, M. (1998). Mentalization and the changing aims of child psychoanalysis. *Psychoanalytic Dialogues, 8,* 87–114.

Foreman, S. A., & Marmar, C. R. (1985). Therapist actions that address initially poor therapeutic alliances in psychotherapy. *American Journal of Psychiatry, 142,* 922–926.

Freud, A. (1936). *The ego and mechanisms of defense.* New York: International Universities Press.

Freud, S. (1910/1957). The future prospects of psycho-analytic therapy. In *Standard edition* (Vol. 11, pp. 139–151). London: Hogarth Press.

Freud, S. (1912/1958). The dynamics of transference. In *Standard edition* (Vol. 12, pp. 97–108). London: Hogarth Press.

Freud, S. (1917/1963). Mourning and melancholia. In *Standard edition* (Vol. 14, pp. 237–260). London: Hogarth Press.

Freud, S. (1923/1961). The ego and the id. In *Standard edition* (Vol. 19, pp. 1–66). London: Hogarth Press.

Freud, S. (1937/1964). Analysis terminable and interminable. *Standard edition* (Vol. 23, pp. 209–253). London: Hogarth Press.

Freud, S. (1940/1964). An outline of psycho-analysis. In *Standard edition* (Vol. 23, pp. 139–207). London: Hogarth Press.

Friedman, L. (1969). The therapeutic alliance. *International Journal of Psycho-Analysis, 50,* 139–153.

Friedman, L. (1988). *The anatomy of psychotherapy.* Hillsdale, NJ: Analytic Press.

Frijda, N. H. (1986). *The emotions.* New York: Cambridge University Press.

Fromm, E. (1947). *A man for himself.* New York: Rinehart.

Fromm, E. (1964). *The heart of man.* New York: Harper & Row.

Gabbard, G. C. (1995). Countertransference: The emerging common ground. *International Journal of Psycho-Analysis, 76,* 475–486.

Gabbard, G. O. (1996). *Love and hate in the analytic setting.* Northvale, NJ: Aronson.

Gabbard, G. O., & Wilkinson, S. M. (1994). *Management of countertransference with borderline patients.* Washington, DC: American Psychiatric Press.

Gadamer, H.-G. (1960/1975). *Truth and method* (trans. and ed. G. Barden & J. Cumming). New York: Seabury Press.

Gaston, L. (1990). The concept of the alliance and its role in psychotherapy: Theoretical and empirical considerations. *Psychotherapy: Theory, Research, and Practice, 27,* 143–153.

Gendlin, E. (1968). Client-centered: The experiential response. In E. F. Hammer (ed.), *The use of interpretation in treatment: Technique and art* (pp. 208–227). New York: Grune & Stratton.

Gendlin, E. T. (1981). *Focusing.* New York: Bantam Books.

Gendlin, E. (1991). On emotion in therapy. In J. D. Safran & L. S. Greenberg (eds.), *Emotion, psychotherapy, and change* (pp. 255–279). New York: Guilford Press.

Gendlin, E. (1994). *Focusing-oriented psychotherapy: A manual of the experiential method.* New York: Guilford Press.

Ghent, E. (1989). Credo: The dialectics of one-person and two-person psychologies. *Contemporary Psychoanalysis, 25,* 169–211.

Ghent, E. (1992). Paradox and process. *Psychoanalytic Dialogues, 2,* 135–160.

Ghent, E. (1993). Wish, need, and neediness: Commentary on Shabad's "Resentment, indignation, and entitlement." *Psychoanalytic Dialogues, 3,* 495–508.

Gibson, J. J. (1979). *The ecological approach to visual perception.* Boston: Houghton Mifflin.

Gill, M. M. (1982). *Analysis of transference: Vol. 1. Theory and technique.* New York: International Universities Press.

Goldfried, M., & Davison, G. (1974). *Clinical behavior therapy.* New York: Holt, Rinehart & Winston.

Goldfried, M., & Davison, G. (1994). *Clinical behavior therapy* (expanded ed.). New York: Wiley.

Gray, P. (1994). *The ego and analysis of defense*. Northvale, NJ: Aronson.

Greenacre, P. (1968). The psychoanalytic process, transference, and acting out. *International Journal of Psycho-Analysis, 49,* 211–218.

Greenberg, J. (1986). Theoretical models and the analyst's neutrality. *Contemporary Psychoanalysis, 22,* 87–106.

Greenberg, J. (1991). *Oedipus and beyond.* Cambridge, MA: Harvard University Press.

Greenberg, J. (1995). Psychoanalytic technique and the interactive matrix. *Psychoanalytic Quarterly, 64,* 1–22.

Greenberg, J. (1999). *The analyst's participation: A fresh look.* The Bernard Kalinkowitz lecture, New York University postdoctoral program in psychotherapy and psychoanalysis.

Greenberg, J., & Mitchell, S. A. (1983). *Object relations in psychoanalytic theory.* Cambridge, MA: Harvard University Press.

Greenberg, L. S. (1986). Change process research. *Journal of Consulting and Clinical Psychology, 54,* 4–11.

Greenberg, L. S., Rice, L. N., & Elliott, R. (1993). *Facilitating emotional change: The moment-by-moment process.* New York: Guilford Press.

Greenberg, L. S., & Safran, J. D. (1987). *Emotion in psychotherapy.* New York: Guilford Press.

Greenson, R. (1967). *The technique and practice of psychoanalysis.* New York: International Universities Press.

Greenson, R. (1971). The real relationship between the patient and the psychoanalyst. In M. Kanzer (ed.), *The unconscious today* (pp. 213–232). New York: International Universities Press.

Greenson, R. (1974). Transference: Freud or Klein? *International Journal of Psycho-Analysis, 55,* 37–48.

Guidano, V. F. (1987). *Complexity of the self.* New York: Guilford Press.

Guidano, V. F. (1991). *The self in process.* New York: Guilford Press.

Guntrip, H. I. (1969). *Schizoid phenomena, object relations, and the self.* New York: International Universities Press.

Gutheil, T. G., & Havens, L. L. (1979). The therapeutic alliance: Contemporary meanings and confusions. *Review of Psychoanalysis, 6,* 467–481.

Habermas, J. (1971). *Knowledge and human interests* (trans. J. Shapiro). Boston: Beacon Press.

Habermas, J. (1987). *The theory of communicative action* (trans. T. McCarthy). Boston: Beacon Press.

Hanly, C. (1992). Reflections on the place of the therapeutic alliance in psychoanalysis. *International Journal of Psycho-Analysis, 75,* 457–467.

Harper, H. (1989a). *Coding Guide I: Identification of confrontation challenges in exploratory therapy.* University of Sheffield, Sheffield, England.

Harper, H. (1989b). *Coding Guide II: Identification of withdrawal challenges in exploratory therapy.* University of Sheffield, Sheffield, England.

Hartley, D. E. (1985). Research on the therapeutic alliance in psychotherapy. In

R. Hales & A. Frances (eds.), *Psychiatry update* (pp. 532–549). Washington, DC: American Psychiatric Association Press.

Hartmann, H. (1958). *Ego psychology and the problem of adaptation.* New York: International Universities Press.

Haynal, A. (1989). *Controversies in psychoanalytic method.* New York: New York University Press.

Hegel, G. W. F. (1807/1977). *Phenomenology of spirit* (trans. A. V. Miller). London: Oxford University Press.

Heimann, P. (1950). On transference. *International Journal of Psycho-Analysis, 31,* 81–84.

Heimberg, R. (1998). Manual-based treatment: An essential ingredient of clinical practice in the 21st century. *Clinical Psychology: Science and Practice, 5,* 387–390.

Henry, W. P. (1998). Science, politics, and the politics of science: The use and misuse of empirically validated treatment research. *Psychotherapy Research, 8,* 126–140.

Henry, W. P., Schacht, T. E., & Strupp, H. H. (1986). Structural analysis of social behavior: Application to a study of interpersonal process in differential psychotherapeutic outcome. *Journal of Consulting and Clinical Psychology, 54,* 27–31.

Henry, W. P., Schacht, T. E., & Strupp, H. H. (1990). Patient and therapist introjects, interpersonal process and differential psychotherapy outcome. *Journal of Consulting and Clinical Psychology, 58,* 768–774.

Henry, W. P., Schacht, T. E., Strupp, H. H., Butler, S. F., & Binder, J. L. (1993). Effects of training in time-limited dynamic psychotherapy: Mediators of therapists' responses to training. *Journal of Consulting and Clinical Psychology, 61,* 441–447.

Henry, W. P., & Strupp, H. H. (1994). The therapeutic alliance as interpersonal process. In A. O. Horvath & L. S. Greenberg (eds.), *The working alliance: Theory, research, and practice* (pp. 51–84). New York: Wiley.

Henry, W. P., Strupp, H. H., Butler, S. F., Schacht, T. E., & Binder, J. L. (1993). Effects of training in time-limited psychotherapy: Changes in therapist behavior. *Journal of Consulting and Clinical Psychology, 61,* 434–440.

Hidas, G. (1993). Flowing over-transference, countertransference, telepathy: Subjective dimensions of the psychoanalytic relationship in Ferenczi's thinking. In L. Aron & A. Harris (eds.), *The legacy of Sandor Ferenczi* (pp. 207–216). Hillsdale, NJ: Analytic Press.

Hirsch, I. (1996). Observing participation, mutual enactment, and the new classical models. *Contemporary Psychoanalysis, 32,* 359–383.

Hoffman, I. Z. (1994). Dialectic thinking and therapeutic action in the psychoanalytic process. *Psychoanalytic Quarterly, 63,* 187–218.

Hoffman, I. Z. (1998). *Ritual and spontaneity in the psychoanalytic process: A dialectical–constructivist view.* Hillsdale, NJ: Analytic Press.

Holton, G. (1971). On trying to understand scientific genius. *American Scholar, 41,* 98–99.

Horney, K. (1950). *Neurosis and human growth.* New York: Norton.

Horowitz, M. J. (1987). *States of mind* (2d ed.). New York: Plenum Press.

Horowitz, M. J. (1991). Short-term dynamic therapy of stress response syndromes. In P. Crits-Christoph & J. P. Barber (eds.), *Handbook of short-term dynamic psychotherapy* (pp. 166–198). New York: Basic Books.

Horvath, A. O. (1995). The therapeutic relationship: From transference to alliance. *In Session: Psychotherapy in Practice, 1,* 7–18.

Horvath, A. O., Gaston, L., & Luborsky, L. (1993). The therapeutic alliance and its measures. In N. Miller, L. Luborsky, J. Barber, & J. Docherty (eds.), *Handbook of psychodynamic psychotherapy: Theory and research* (pp. 247–273). New York: Basic Books.

Horvath, A. O., & Greenberg, L. S. (1989). Development and validation of the Working Alliance Inventory. *Journal of Counseling Psychology, 36,* 223–233.

Horvath, A. O., & Greenberg, L. S., eds. (1994). *The working alliance: Theory, research, and practice.* New York: Wiley.

Horvath, A. O., & Luborsky, L. (1993). The role of the therapeutic alliance in psychotherapy. *Journal of Consulting and Clinical Psychology, 61,* 561–573.

Horvath, A. O., & Symonds, B. D. (1991). Relation between working alliance and outcome in psychotherapy: A meta-analysis. *Journal of Counseling Psychology, 38,* 139–149.

Jacobs, T. (1986). On countertransference enactments. *Journal of the American Psychoanalytic Association, 34,* 289–307.

Jacobs, T. (1991). *The use of the self: Countertransference and communication in the analytic setting.* Madison, CT: International Universities Press.

James, W. (1890/1981). *The principles of psychology.* Cambridge, MA: Harvard University Press.

Jones, J. M. (1995). *Affects as process: An inquiry into the centrality of affect in psychological life.* Hillsdale, NJ: Analytic Press.

Joseph, B. (1989). *Psychic equilibrium and psychic change* (ed. M. Feldman & E. B. Spillius). London and New York: Tavistock and Routledge.

Kabat-Zinn, J. (1991). *Full catastrophe living.* New York: Delta.

Kaiser, H. (1965). *The problem of responsibility in psychotherapy* (ed. L. B. Fierman). New York: Free Press.

Kanzer, M. (1975). The therapeutic and working alliances: An assessment. *International Journal of Psychoanalytic Psychotherapy, 4,* 48–68.

Kennedy, R. (1997). On subjective organizations: Toward a theory of subject relations. *Psychoanalytic Dialogues, 7,* 553–581.

Kernberg, O. F. (1965). Notes on countertransference. *Journal of the American Psychoanalytic Association, 13,* 38–56.

Kiesler, D. J. (1996). *Contemporary interpersonal theory and research: Personality, psychopathology, and psychotherapy.* New York: Wiley.

Kiesler, D. J., & Watkins, K. (1989). Interpersonal complementarity and the therapeutic alliance: A study of relationship in psychotherapy. *Psychotherapy: Theory, Research, and Practice, 26,* 183–194.

Klein, M. (1975). *"Envy and gratitude" and other works, 1946–1963.* New York: Delacorte.

Klerman, G., Weissman, M., Rounsaville, B., & Chevron, E. (1984). *Interpersonal psychotherapy for depression.* New York: Basic Books.

Kohlenberg, R., & Tsai, M. (1991). *Functional analytic psychotherapy*. New York: Plenum Press.

Kohut, H. (1971). *The analysis of the self*. New York: International Universities Press.

Kohut, H. (1977). *The restoration of the self*. New York: International Universities Press.

Kohut, H. (1984). *How does analysis cure?* Chicago: University of Chicago Press.

Korzybski, A. (1933). *Science and sanity*. San Francisco: International Society of General Semantics.

Kris, E. (1951). Ego psychology and interpretation in psychoanalytic therapy. *Psychoanalytic Quarterly, 20*, 15–30.

Lacan, J. (1953/1977). *Ecrits: A selection* (trans. A. Sheridan). New York: Norton.

Lacan, J. (1973a/1988). *The seminar of Jacques Lacan: Book 1. Freud's papers on technique, 1953–1954* (trans. A. Sheridan). New York: Norton.

Lacan, J. (1973b/1988). *The seminar of Jacques Lacan: Book 2. The ego in Freud's theory and in the technique of psychoanalysis, 1954–1955* (trans. A. Sheridan). New York: Norton.

Laing, R. D. (1969). *Self and others*. New York: Pantheon Books.

Lambert, M. (1998). Manual-based treatment and clinical practice: Hangman of life or promising development? *Clinical Psychology: Science and Practice, 5*, 391–395.

Lang, P. J. (1983). Cognition and emotion: Concept and action. In C. Izard, J. Kagan, & R. Zajonc (eds.), *Emotion, cognition, and behavior* (pp. 192–226). New York: Cambridge University Press.

Langs, R. (1976). *The therapeutic interaction* (2 vols.). Northvale, NJ: Aronson.

Levenson, E. (1972). *The fallacy of understanding*. New York: Basic Books.

Levenson, E. (1983). *The ambiguity of change*. New York: Basic Books.

Levenson, E. (1992). *The purloined self: Interpersonal perspectives in psychoanalysis*. New York: Contemporary Psychoanalysis Books.

Levenson, E. (1998). Awareness, insight, and learning. *Contemporary Psychoanalysis, 34*, 239–250.

Levenson, H. (1995). *Time-limited dynamic psychotherapy: A guide to clinical practice*. New York: Basic Books.

Leventhal, H. (1984). A perceptual–motor theory of emotion. In L. Berkowitz (ed.), *Advances in experimental social psychology* (pp. 117–182). New York: Academic Press.

Lichtenberg, J. (1989). *Psychoanalysis and motivation*. Hillsdale, NJ: Analytic Press.

Lichtenberg, J., Lachmann, F., & Fosshage, J. (1992). *Self and motivational systems: Toward a theory of psychoanalytic technique*. Hillsdale, NJ: Analytic Press.

Linehan, M. (1992). *Cognitive–behavioral treatment of borderline personality disorder*. New York: Guilford Press.

Lionells, M., Fiscalini, J., Mann, C. H., & Stern, D. B., eds. (1995). *The handbook of interpersonal psychoanalysis*. Hillsdale, NJ: Analytic Press.

Liotti, G. (1987). The resistance to change of cognitive structures: A counterproposal to psychoanalytic metapsychology. *Journal of Cognitive Psychotherapy, 2*, 87–104.

Little, M. (1951). Countertransference and the patient's response to it. *International Journal of Psycho-Analysis, 32*, 32–40.

Luborsky, L. (1976). Helping alliances in psychotherapy. In J. L. Claghorn (ed.), *Successful psychotherapy* (pp. 92–116). New York: Brunner/Mazel.

Luborsky, L. (1984). *Principles of psychoanalytic psychotherapy: A manual for supportive-expressive treatment.* New York: Basic Books.

Luborsky, L., & DeRubeis, R. (1984). The use of psychotherapy treatment manuals: A small revolution in psychotherapy research style. *Clinical Psychology Review, 4,* 5–14.

Luborsky, L., McLellan, A. T., Diguer, L., Woody, G., & Seligman, D. A. (1997). The psychotherapist matters: Comparison of outcomes across twenty-two therapists and seven patient samples. *Clinical Psychology: Science and Practice, 4,* 53–65.

MacKenzie, K. R. (1998). The alliance in time-limited group psychotherapy. In J. D. Safran & J. C. Muran (eds.), *The therapeutic alliance in brief psychotherapy* (pp. 193–216). Washington, DC: American Psychological Association Books.

Mahler, M. (1968). *On human symbiosis and the vicissitudes of individuation.* New York: International Universities Press.

Mahoney, M. J. (1991). *Human change processes.* New York: Basic Books.

Malan, D. H. (1963). *A study of brief psychotherapy.* New York: Plenum Press.

Mann, J. (1973). *Time-limited psychotherapy.* Cambridge, MA: Harvard University Press.

Maroda, K. J. (1991/1995). *The power of countertransference: Innovations in analytic technique.* New York: Wiley. (2d ed. Northvale, NJ: Aronson)

McLaughlin, J. T. (1991). Clinical and theoretical aspects of enactment. *Journal of the American Psychoanalytic Association, 39,* 595–614.

Meissner, W. W. (1996). *The therapeutic alliance.* New Haven, CT: Yale University Press.

Messer, S. B., & Warren, C. S. (1995). *Models of brief psychotherapy.* New York: Guilford Press.

Minuchin, S., & Fishman, H. C. (1981). *Family therapy techniques.* Cambridge, MA: Harvard University Press.

Mitchell, S. A. (1988). *Relational concepts in psychoanalysis.* Cambridge, MA: Harvard University Press.

Mitchell, S. A. (1992). True selves, false selves, and the ambiguity of authenticity. In N. J. Skolnick & S. C. Warshaw (eds.), *Relational perspectives in psychoanalysis* (pp. 1–20). Hillsdale, NJ: Analytic Press.

Mitchell, S. A. (1993). *Hope and dread in psychoanalysis.* New York: Basic Books.

Mitchell, S. A. (1997). *Influence and autonomy in psychoanalysis.* Hillsdale, NJ: Analytic Press.

Modell, A. H. (1991). A confusion of tongues or whose reality is it? *Psychoanalytic Quarterly, 60,* 227–244.

Moncher, F. J., & Prinz, R. J. (1991). Treatment fidelity in outcome studies. *Clinical Psychology Review 11,* 247–266.

Money-Kyrle, R. (1956). Normal counter-transference and some of its deviations. *International Journal of Psycho-Analysis, 37,* 360–366.

Muran, J. C. (1993). The self in cognitive behavioral research: An interpersonal perspective. *Behavior Therapist, 16,* 69–73.

Muran, J. C. (1997). Multiple selves and depression. *In session: Psychotherapy in Practice, 3*, 53–64.

Muran, J. C. (in press). Meditations on "both/and." In J. C. Muran (ed.), *Self-relations in the psychotherapy process*. Washington, DC: American Psychological Association Books.

Muran, J. C., Gorman, B., Safran, J. D., Twining, L., Samstag, L. W., & Winston, A. (1995). Linking in-session change to overall outcome in short-term cognitive therapy. *Journal of Consulting and Clinical Psychology, 63*, 651–657.

Muran, J. C., Samstag, L. W., Segal, Z. V., & Winston, A. (1998). Interpersonal scenarios: An idiographic measure of self-schemas. *Psychotherapy Research, 8*, 321–333.

Muran, J. C., Segal, Z. V., Samstag, L. W., & Crawford, C. (1994). Patient pretreatment interpersonal problems and therapeutic alliance in short-term cognitive therapy. *Journal of Consulting and Clinical Psychology, 62*, 185–190.

Muran, J. C., & Ventur, E. (1995). The operent self. *The Behavior Therapist, 18*, 91–94.

Natterson, J. (1991). *Beyond countertransference*. Northvale, NJ: Aronson.

Newirth, J. (1995). Impasses in the psychoanalytic relationship. *In Session: Psychotherapy in Practice, 1*, 73–80.

Newman, C. (1998). The therapeutic relationship and alliance in short-term cognitive therapy. In J. D. Safran & J. C. Muran (eds.), *The therapeutic alliance in brief psychotherapy* (pp. 95–122). Washington, DC: American Psychological Association Books.

Ogden, T. (1979). On projective identification. *International Journal of Psycho-Analysis, 60*, 357–373.

Ogden, T. (1982). *Projective identification and psychotherapeutic technique*. New York: Aronson.

Ogden, T. (1986). *The matrix of the mind*. Northvale, NJ: Aronson.

Ogden, T. (1994). *Subjects of analysis*. Northvale, NJ: Aronson.

Orlinsky, D. A., Grawe, K., & Parks, B. K. (1994). Process and outcome in psychotherapy: Noch einmal. In A. E. Bergin & S. L. Garfield (eds.), *Handbook of psychotherapy and behavior change* (4th ed., pp. 270–376). New York: Wiley.

Parkinson, B. (1995). *Ideas and realities of emotion*. London: Routledge.

Perls, F. (1973). *The gestalt approach and eyewitness therapy*. Palo Alto, CA: Science and Behavior Books.

Pinsof, W., & Catherall, D. (1986). The integrative psychotherapy alliance: Family, couple, and individual therapy scales. *Journal of Marital and Family Therapy, 12*, 137–151.

Pizer, S. A. (1992). The negotiation of paradox in the analytic process. *Psychoanalytic Dialogues, 2*, 215–240.

Pizer, S. A. (1996). The distributed self: Introduction to symposium on "The Multiplicity of Self and Analytic Technique." *Contemporary Psychoanalysis, 32*, 499–507.

Pizer, S. A. (1998). *Building bridges: The negotiation of paradox in psychoanalysis*. Hillsdale, NJ: Analytic Press.

Plutchik, R., & Conte, H., eds. (1997). *Circumplex models of personality and emotion*. Washington, DC: American Psychological Association Books.

Polanyi, M. (1966). *The tacit dimension*. New York: Doubleday.

Racker, H. (1953). A contribution to the problem of countertransference. *International Journal of Psycho-Analysis, 43*, 313–324.

Racker, H. (1968). *Transference and countertransference*. New York: International Universities Press.

Rait, D. (1998). Perspectives on the therapeutic alliance in brief couple and family therapy. In J. D. Safran & J. C. Muran (eds.), *The therapeutic alliance in brief psychotherapy* (pp. 171–191). Washington, DC: American Psychological Association Books.

Rank, O. (1929). *The trauma of birth*. New York: Harcourt, Brace.

Rank, O. (1945). *Will therapy and truth and reality*. New York: Knopf.

Reich, W. (1949). *Character analysis*. New York: Orgone Institute Press.

Reik, T. (1948). *Listening with the third ear: The inner experience of a psychoanalyst*. New York: Farrar, Straus & Giroux.

Renik, O. (1993). Analytic interaction: Conceptualizing technique in light of the analyst's irreducible subjectivity. *Psychoanalytic Quarterly, 62*, 553–571.

Renik, O. (1995). The ideal of the anonymous analyst and the problem of self-disclosure. *Psychoanalytic Quarterly, 64*, 466–495.

Renik, O. (1996). The perils of neutrality. *Psychoanalytic Quarterly, 65*, 495–517.

Renik, O. (1998). The role of countertransference enactment in a successful clinical psychoanalysis. In S. J. Ellman & M. Moskowitz (eds.), *Enactment: Toward a new approach to the therapeutic relationship* (pp. 111–128). Northvale, NJ: Aronson.

Rhodes, R., Hill, C., Thompson, B., & Elliott, R. (1994). Client retrospective recall of resolved and unresolved misunderstanding events. *Counseling Psychology, 41*, 473–483.

Rice, L. N., & Greenberg, L. S. (1984). *Patterns of change*. New York: Guilford Press.

Rock, M., ed. (1997). *Psychodynamic supervision*. Northvale, NJ: Aronson.

Rogers, C. R. (1951). *Client-centered therapy*. Boston: Houghton Mifflin.

Rogers, C. R. (1957). The necessary and sufficient conditions of therapeutic personality change. *Journal of Consulting Psychology, 21*, 95–103.

Rosch, E. (1988). Principles of categorization. In A. M. Collins & E. E. Smith (eds.), *Readings in cognitive science: A perspective from psychology and artificial intelligence* (pp. 312–322). San Matteo, CA: Kaufmann.

Rubin, J. R. (1996). *Psychotherapy and Buddhism: Towards an integration*. New York: Plenum Press.

Safran, J. D. (1984a). Assessing the cognitive–interpersonal cycle. *Cognitive Therapy and Research, 8*, 333–348.

Safran, J. D. (1984b). Some implications of Sullivan's interpersonal theory for cognitive therapy. In M. A. Reda & M. J. Mahoney (eds.), *Cognitive psychotherapies: Recent developments in theory, research and practice*. Cambridge, MA: Ballinger.

Safran, J. D. (1990a). Towards a refinement of cognitive therapy in light of interpersonal theory: I. Theory. *Clinical Psychology Review, 10*, 87–105.

Safran, J. D. (1990b). Towards a refinement of cognitive therapy in light of interpersonal theory: II. Practice. *Clinical Psychology Review, 10*, 107–121.

Safran, J. D. (1993a). Breaches in the therapeutic alliance: An arena for negotiating authentic relatedness. *Psychotherapy: Theory, Research, and Practice, 30*, 11–24.

Safran, J. D. (1993b). The therapeutic alliance as a transtheoretical phenomenon: Definitional and conceptual issues. *Journal of Psychotherapy Integration, 3*, 33–49.

Safran, J. D. (1998). *Widening the scope of cognitive therapy*. Northvale, NJ: Aronson.

Safran, J. D. (1999). Faith, despair, will, and the paradox of acceptance. *Contemporary Psychoanalysis, 35*, 5–24.

Safran, J. D. (in press). Brief relational psychoanalytic treatment. *Psychoanalytic Dialogues*.

Safran, J. D., Crocker, P., McMain, S., & Murray, P. (1990). Therapeutic alliance rupture as a therapy event for empirical investigation. *Psychotherapy: Theory, Research, and Practice, 27*, 154–165.

Safran, J. D., & Greenberg, L. S., eds. (1991). *Emotion, psychotherapy, and change*. New York: Guilford Press.

Safran, J. D., Greenberg, L. S., & Rice, L. N. (1988). Integrating psychotherapy research and practice: Modeling the change process. *Psychotherapy: Theory, Research, and Practice, 25*, 1–17.

Safran, J. D., & Muran, J. C. (1994). Toward a working alliance between research and practice. In P. F. Talley, H. H. Strupp, & S. F. Butler (eds.), *Psychotherapy research and practice: Bridging the gap* (pp. 206–226). New York: Basic Books.

Safran, J. D., & Muran, J. C. (1995). Resolving therapeutic alliance ruptures: Diversity and integration. *In Session: Psychotherapy in Practice, 1*, 81–82.

Safran, J. D., & Muran, J. C. (1996). The resolution of ruptures in the therapeutic alliance. *Journal of Consulting and Clinical Psychology, 64*, 447–458.

Safran, J. D., & Muran, J. C., eds. (1998). *The therapeutic alliance in brief psychotherapy*. Washington, DC: American Psychological Association Books.

Safran, J. D., Muran, J. C., & Samstag, L. W. (1994). Resolving therapeutic alliance ruptures: A task analytic investigation. In A. O. Horvath & L. S. Greenberg (eds.), *The working alliance: Theory, research, and practice* (pp. 225–255). New York: Wiley.

Safran, J. D., & Segal, Z. V. (1990/1996). *Interpersonal process in cognitive therapy*. New York: Basic Books. (2d ed. Northvale, NJ: Aronson)

Safran, J. D., & Wallner, L. (1991). The relative predictive validity of two therapeutic alliance measures in cognitive therapy. *Psychological Assessment: A Journal of Consulting and Clinical Psychology, 3*, 188–195.

Sandler, J. (1976). Countertransference and role-responsiveness. *International Journal of Psycho-Analysis, 3*, 43–47.

Sandler, J., Dare, C., & Holder, A. (1992). *The patient and the analyst: The basis of the psychoanalytic process* (2d ed.). Madison, CT: International Universities Press.

Sandler, J., Holder, A., Kawenoka, M., Kennedy, H., & Neurath, L. (1969). Notes on some theoretical and clinical aspects of transference. *International Journal of Psycho-Analysis, 50*, 633–645.

Sartre, J.-P. (1943/1956). *Being and nothingness* (trans. H. E. Barnes). New York: Washington Square Press.

Schachtel, E. (1959). *Metamorphisis*. New York: Basic Books.

Schafer, R. (1983). *The analytic attitude*. New York: Basic Books.

Schafer, R. (1992). *Retelling a life: Narration and dialogue in psychoanalysis*. New York: Basic Books.

Schon, D. (1983). *The reflexive practitioner.* New York: Basic Books.

Searles, H. (1955). The informational value of the supervisor's emotional experience. *Psychiatry, 18,* 135–146.

Searles, H. (1979). *Countertransference and related subjects.* New York: International Universities Press.

Seligman, M. (1995). The effectiveness of psychotherapy. *American Psychologist, 50,* 965–974.

Seligman, S. (1999). Integrating Kleinian theory and intersubjective infant research: Observing projective identification. *Psychoanalytic Dialogues, 9,* 129–160.

Shabad, P. (1993). Resentment, indignation, entitlement: The transformation of unconscious wish into need. *Psychoanalytic Quarterly, 3,* 481–494.

Shapiro, D. (1965). *Neurotic styles.* New York: Basic Books.

Shapiro, D. (1989). *Psychotherapy of neurotic character.* New York: Basic Books.

Shaw, R., & Bransford, J., eds. (1977). *Perceiving, acting, and knowing: Toward an ecological psychology.* Hillsdale, NJ: Erlbaum.

Sifneos, P. E. (1972). *Short-term psychotherapy and emotional crisis.* Cambridge, MA: Harvard University Press.

Singer, E. (1977). *Key concepts in psychotherapy.* Northvale, NJ: Aronson.

Slochower, J. (1996). Holding and the fate of the analyst's subjectivity. *Psychoanalytic Dialogues, 6,* 323–354.

Slochower, J. (1997). *Holding and psychoanalysis.* Hillsdale, NJ: Analytic Press.

Smith, M. L., Glass, G. V., & Miller, M. I. (1980). *The benefits of psychotherapy.* Baltimore: Johns Hopkins University Press.

Spezzano, C. (1993). *Affect in psychoanalysis.* Hillsdale, NJ: Analytic Press.

Spezzano, C. (1998). The triangle of clinical judgment. *Journal of the American Psychoanalytic Association, 46,* 365–388.

Stanton, M. (1990). *Sandor Ferenczi: Reconsidering active intervention.* London: Free Press.

Sterba, R. (1934). The fate of the ego in analytic therapy. *International Journal of Psycho-Analysis, 15,* 117–126.

Sterba, R. (1940). The dynamics of the dissolution of the transference resistance. *Psychoanalytic Quarterly, 9,* 363–379.

Stern, D. N. (1985). *The interpersonal world of the infant.* New York: Basic Books.

Stern, D. B. (1997). *Unformulated experience.* Hillsdale, NJ: Analytic Press.

Stolorow, R., & Atwood, G. (1992). *Contexts of being: The intersubjective foundations of psychological life.* Hillsdale, NJ: Analytic Press.

Stolorow, R., Brandchaft, B., & Atwood, G. (1994). *Psychoanalytic treatment: An intersubjective approach.* Hillsdale, NJ: Analytic Press.

Stone, L. (1961). *The psychoanalytic situation.* New York: International Universities Press.

Strachey, J. (1934). The nature of the therapeutic action of psychoanalysis. *International Journal of Psycho-Analysis, 15,* 127–159.

Strupp, H. H. (1993). The Vanderbilt Psychotherapy Studies: Synopsis. *Journal of Consulting and Clinical Psychology, 61,* 431–433.

Strupp, H. H., & Anderson, T. (1997). On the limitations of treatment manuals. *Clinical Psychology: Science and Practice, 4,* 76–82.

Strupp, H. H., & Binder, J. L. (1984). *Psychotherapy in a new key: A guide to time-limited dynamic psychotherapy*. New York: Basic Books.

Strupp, H. H., Butler, S. F., & Rosser, C. L. (1988). Training in psychodynamic therapy. *Journal of Consulting and Clinical Psychology, 56,* 669–689.

Sullivan, H. S. (1953). *The interpersonal theory of psychiatry*. New York: Norton.

Sullivan, H. S. (1954). *The psychiatric interview*. New York: Norton.

Sullivan, H. S. (1956). *Clinical studies in psychiatry*. New York: Norton.

Sullivan, H. S. (1965). *The fusion of psychiatry and the social sciences*. New York: Norton.

Suzuki, S. (1970). *Zen mind, beginner's mind*. New York: Weatherhill.

Symington, N. (1983). The analyst's act of freedom as an agent of therapeutic change. *International Review of Psycho-Analysis, 10,* 783–792.

Tansey, M., & Burke, W. (1989). *Understanding countertransference: From projective identification to empathy*. Hillsdale, NJ: Analytic Press.

Tasca, G. A., & McMullen, L. M. (1992). Interpersonal complementarity and antitheses within a stage model of psychotherapy. *Psychotherapy: Theory, Research, and Practice, 29,* 515–523.

Thompson, C. (1944). Ferenczi's contribution to psychoanalysis. *Psychiatry, 7,* 245–252.

Thompson, C. (1950). *Psychoanalysis: Evolution and development*. New York: Grove Atlantic Monthly Press.

Thompson, C. (1964). *Interpersonal psychoanalysis* (ed. M. Green). New York: Basic Books.

Tomkins, S. S. (1987). Script theory. In V. Aronoff, A. Rabin, & R. Zucker (eds.), *The emergence of personality* (pp. 147–216). New York: Springer-Verlag.

Tronick, E. (1989). Emotions and emotional communications in infants. *American Psychologist, 44,* 112–119.

Varela, F. J., Thompson, E., & Rosch, E. (1991). *The embodied mind: Cognitive science and human experience*. Cambridge, MA: MIT Press.

Wachtel, P. L. (1977). *Psychoanalysis and behavior therapy: Toward an integration*. New York: Basic Books.

Wachtel, P. L. (1993). *Therapeutic communication*. New York: Guilford Press.

Wachtel, P. L. (1997). *Psychoanalysis, behavior therapy, and the relational world*. Washington, DC: American Psychological Association Books.

Wallerstein, R. S. (1995). *The talking cures*. New Haven, CT: Yale University Press.

Watson, J., & Greenberg, L. S. (1995). Alliance ruptures and repairs in experiential therapy. *In Session: Psychotherapy in Practice, 1,* 19–32.

Watzlawick, P. (1978). *The language of change*. New York: Norton.

Watzlawick, P., Beavin, J. H., & Jackson, D. D. (1967). *Pragmatics of human communication*. New York: Norton.

Weimer, W. B. (1977). A conceptual framework for cognitive psychology: Motor theories of the mind. In R. Shaw & J. Bransford (eds.), *Perceiving, acting, and knowing: Toward an ecological psychology* (pp. 267–311). Hillsdale, NJ: Erlbaum.

Weiss, J. (1993). *How psychotherapy works: Process and technique*. New York: Guilford Press.

Weiss, J., Sampson, H., & the Mount Zion Psychotherapy Research Group. (1986).

The psychoanalytic process: Theory, clinical observations, and empirical research. New York: Guilford Press.

Westen, D. (1997). Towards a clinically and empirically sound theory of motivation. *International Journal of Psychoanalysis, 78,* 521–548.

Williams, P. (1989). *Mahayana Buddhism: The doctrinal foundations.* London: Routledge.

Wilner, W. (1975). The nature of intimacy. *Contemporary Psychoanalysis, 11,* 206–226.

Wilson, G. T. (1998). Manual-based treatment and clinical practice. *Clinical Practice: Science and Practice, 5,* 363–375.

Winnicott, D. W. (1947/1958). Hate in the countertransference. In *Through paediatrics to psychoanalysis* (pp. 194–203). New York: Basic Books.

Winnicott, D. W. (1956/1958). Primary maternal preoccupation. In *Through paediatrics to psychoanalysis* (pp. 300–305). New York: Basic Books.

Winnicott, D. W. (1958a). *Through paediatrics to psychoanalysis.* New York: Basic Books.

Winnicott, D. W. (1958b/1965). The capacity to be alone. In *The maturational process and the facilitating environment* (pp. 29–36). New York: International Universities Press.

Winnicott, D. W. (1960/1965). Ego distortion in terms of true and false self. In *The maturational process and the facilitating environment* (pp. 140–152). New York: International Universities Press.

Winnicott, D. W. (1965). *The maturational process and the facilitating environment.* New York: International Universities Press.

Winnicott, D. W. (1969). The use of an object. *International Journal of Psycho-Analysis, 50,* 711–716.

Winnicott, D. W. (1986). *Holding and interpretation.* London: Hogarth Press.

Wolfe, B. E., & Goldfried, M. R. (1988). Research on psychotherapy integration: Recommendations and conclusions from an NIMH workshop. *Journal of Consulting and Clinical Psychology, 56,* 448–451.

Wolstein, B. (1959). *Countertransference.* New York: Grune & Stratton.

Wolstein, B. (1975). Countertransference: The psychoanalyst's shared experience and inquiry with his patient. *Journal of the American Academy of Psychoanalysis, 3,* 77–89.

Wolstein, B. (1988). Introduction. In B. Wolstein (ed.), *Essential papers on countertransference* (pp. 1–15). New York: New York University Press.

Wolstein, B. (1994). The evolving newness of interpersonal psychoanalysis: From the vantage point of immediate experience. *Contemporary Psychoanalysis, 30,* 473–499.

Zetzel, E. (1956). Current concepts of transference. *International Journal of Psycho-Analysis, 37,* 369–375.

Zetzel, E. (1966). The analytic situation. In R. E. Litman (ed.), *Psychoanalysis in America* (pp. 86–106). New York: International Universities Press.

Index